One Minute to a Better Body

77 Shortcuts, Tips and Lessons to Building Muscle Now

From the Editors of

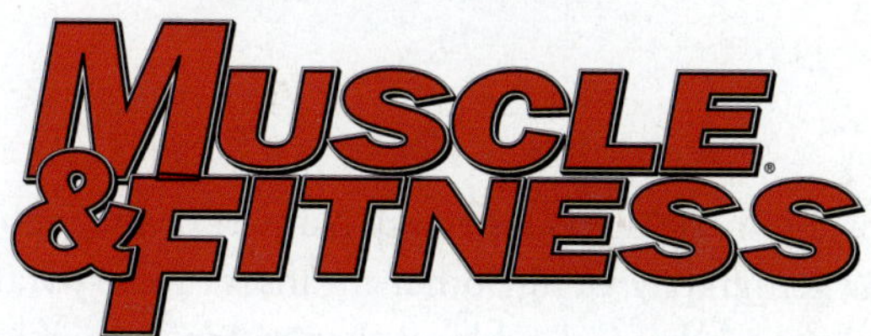

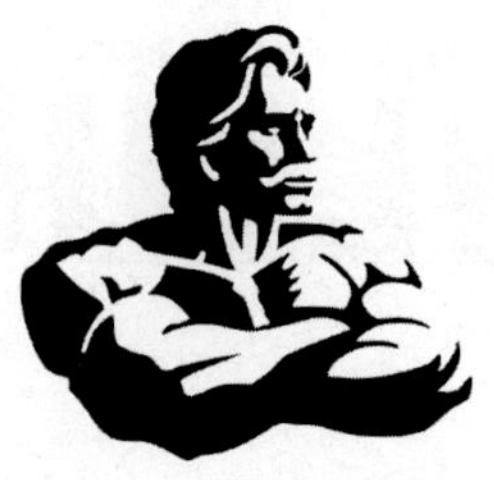

"Strive for excellence, exceed yourself, love your friends, speak the truth, practice fidelity, and honor your father and mother. These principles will help you master yourself, make you strong, give you hope and put you on the path to greatness."

—*Joe Weider,*
Trainer of Champions

ACKNOWLEDGMENTS

This special publication is based on articles written by Timothy C. Fritz, CSCS and Dan Wagman, PhD, CSCS, for MUSCLE & FITNESS magazine. Content in the "Women in the Weight Room" section is based on articles written by Suzanne Meth, MS, ATC, CSCS, Kathleen Engel, and Brian Rowley, MS, for MUSCLE & FITNESS and MUSCLE & FITNESS HERS magazine. Photos by Per Bernal, Chris Lund, Jim Purdin, Roni Ramos, Robert Reiff, Rick Schaff and Cory Sorensen. Illustration by Elaine Kurie. Project and cover design for this book by Kimberly Richey. Project Editor is Jeanine Detz. MUSCLE & FITNESS Executive Editor is Bill Geiger. Editorial assistance provided by Steve Mazzucchi and Joe Wuebben. Photo Editor is Lisa Clark. Photo Archivist is David Marsh. Production Manager is Renee Thompson. Rights and permissions researched by Darlene Salvador. Director of Product Development, Enthusiast Group, is Steven Lombardi. Project Manager, Enthusiast Group, is James Lombardi. Senior Vice President, Group Editorial Director is Vincent Scalisi. Editor in Chief/Group Publisher is Tom Deters, DC. Founder/Publisher is Joe Weider.

CONTENTS

CONTENTS

TIME'S A WASTING

What's 60 seconds to you? About the time it takes you to grab a snack from the kitchen between commercials of the latest reality-based dating show, or perhaps the wait to grab the next elevator to the fifth floor.

If you're fitness-minded, you're thinking it's the time for another lap around the track, or the extra time it takes to walk to the mall entrance because you parked farther away to get in a bit of exercise.

In the gym, there's not much you can do in a minute – maybe an extra set of biceps curls or a nonstop set of crunches. Certainly, 60 seconds isn't the amount of time that's going to make a difference in your workout success, as if that's the magical missing ingredient in your ability to reach those elusive training and physique goals.

While MUSCLE & FITNESS wouldn't be the ones to preach one minute to fitness – we'll leave the 60-second workouts to some of the so-called men's lifestyle magazines that are targeted to those afraid of breaking a sweat — that doesn't mean we're being disingenuous about the title of this book. In fact, each of the 77 topics presented here is a bite-sized golden nugget of training information designed to be read in — you guessed it — about a minute. We compiled them from one of our

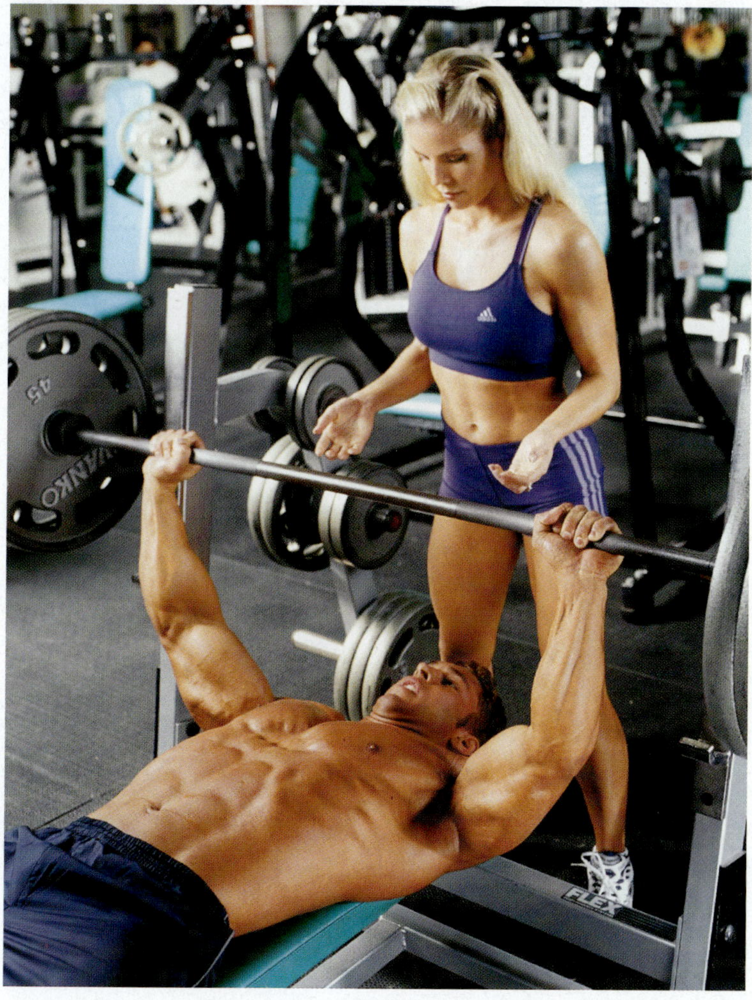

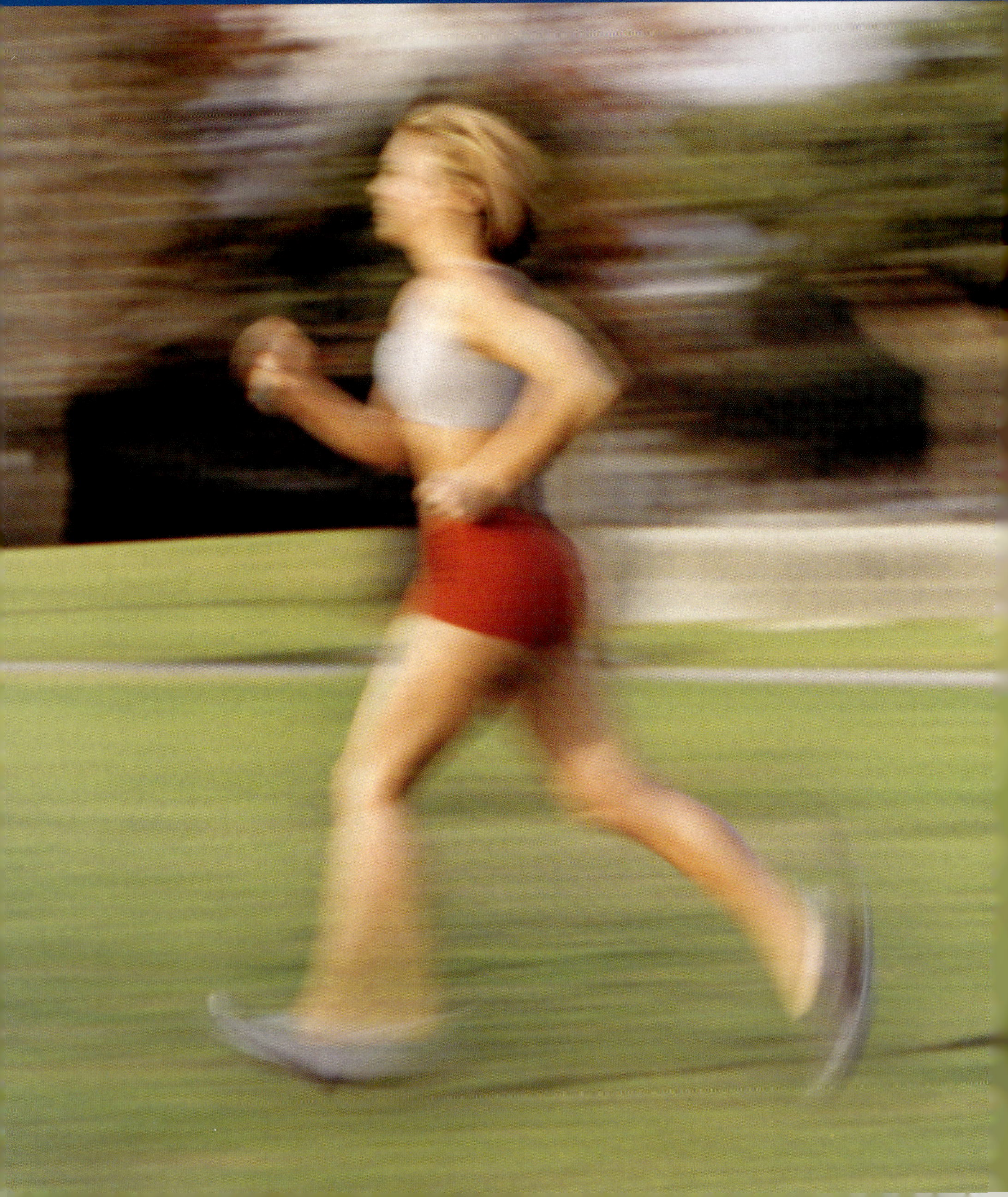

most popular monthly columns in *Muscle & Fitness* — One-Minute Lesson — and arranged them in a meaningful way for ease of navigation through this book, from training theory to specific exercise execution.

What of any significance can you learn in a quick read? Perhaps that's best learned by answering a few short training-related questions:

- When does including machine training make the most sense in your routine?
- Should you change a successful routine?
- What difference does it make when you do an exercise standing vs. seated?
- Is there such thing as a dangerous movement?
- How do you reduce hip-flexor involvement when training abs?
- What's the difference between the pull-up and chin-up?
- Should upright rows be done with back or shoulder training?
- Can you target various areas of the quad when doing leg extensions?
- Does a weight belt improve your performance in the gym?
- Should women train in a different style than men?

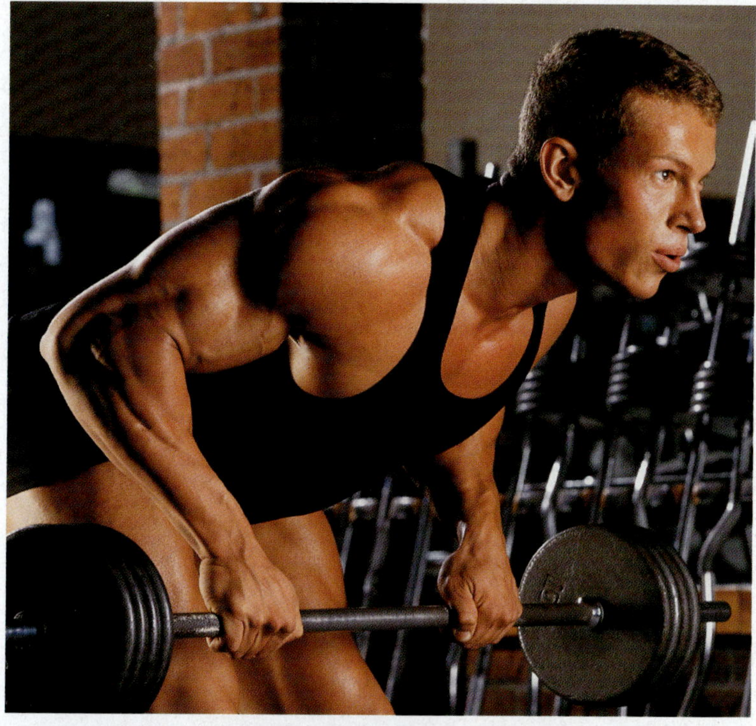

I suspect that even though you know a thing or two about training, you simply don't know why you do certain things in the gym. Perhaps you lock out your elbows on triceps exercises — yes, that can affect your joint health! Maybe you squat with a board under your heels and to a point just short of parallel to the floor — yes, those factors make a real difference! Before hitting the weights, perhaps you stretch first thing — yes, you've got it backward when it comes to warming up! On occasion, maybe you do your cardio session before pumping iron — no, if you want to make your muscles bigger, you're compromising your efforts!

'We tackle some of the most common misconceptions that everyone — from inquisitive beginners to more advanced lifters — makes.'

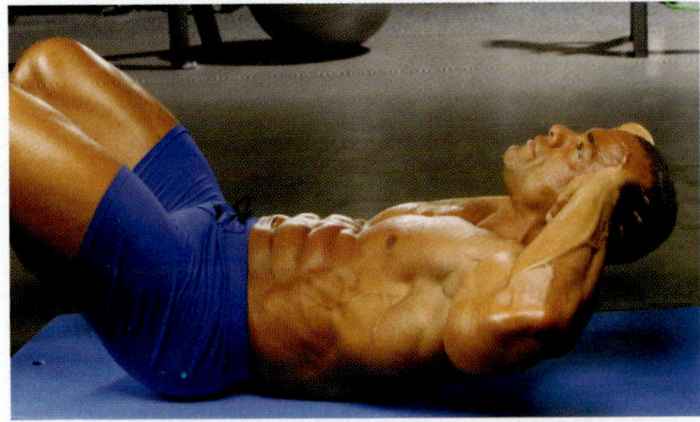

Unlike many how-to exercise books, we've gone beyond providing simple explanations on exercise technique that seem more oriented toward beginners. Instead, we tackle some of the most common misconceptions that everyone — from inquisitive beginners to more advanced lifters — makes, providing a clear explanation that focuses on the why and how. The columns were written by a handful of our top writers, each one not only an experienced gym rat but also certified with the National Strength and Conditioning Association (NSCA), the nation's premier educational organization for certified personal trainers and collegiate and pro strength coaches.

So, in the end, 60 seconds may not be enough to give you that six-pack you've always wanted or increase your bench by 50 pounds, but hopefully it's enough to help you start making faster strides in your training progress. Look around the gym; too many people with the best of intentions spend months making the same mistakes over and over again and have little to show for it. You aren't like them because you've made this investment in improving yourself by training smarter. So let's get started. Time's a wasting.

Bill Geiger
Executive Editor,
MUSCLE & FITNESS

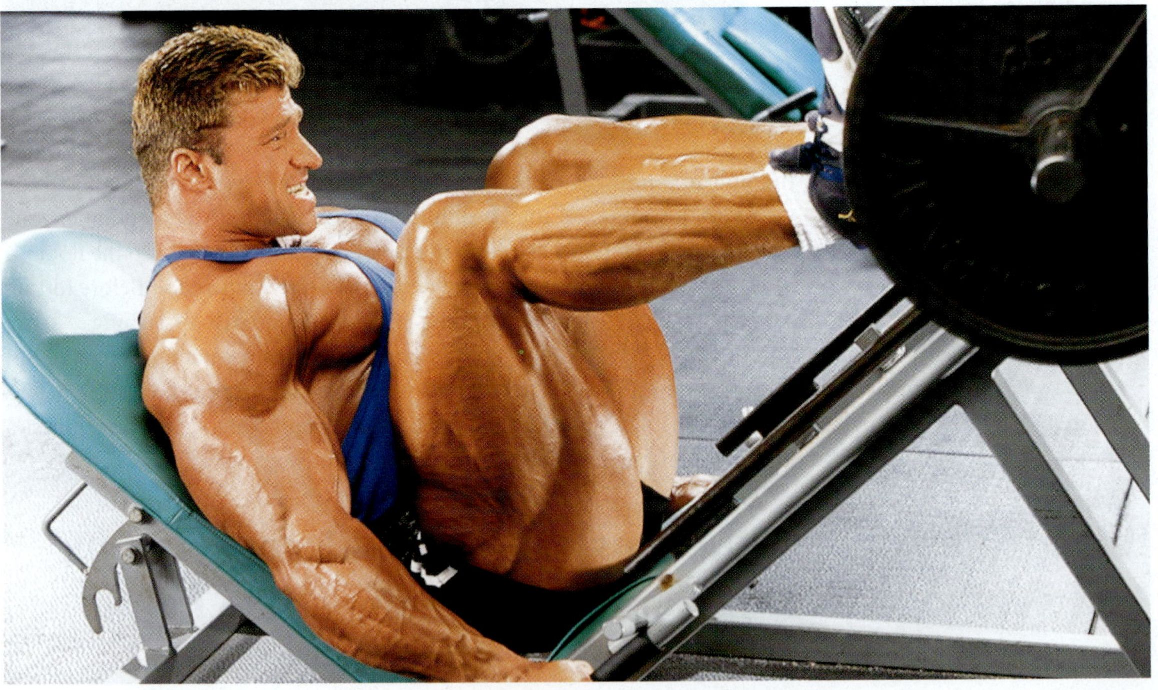

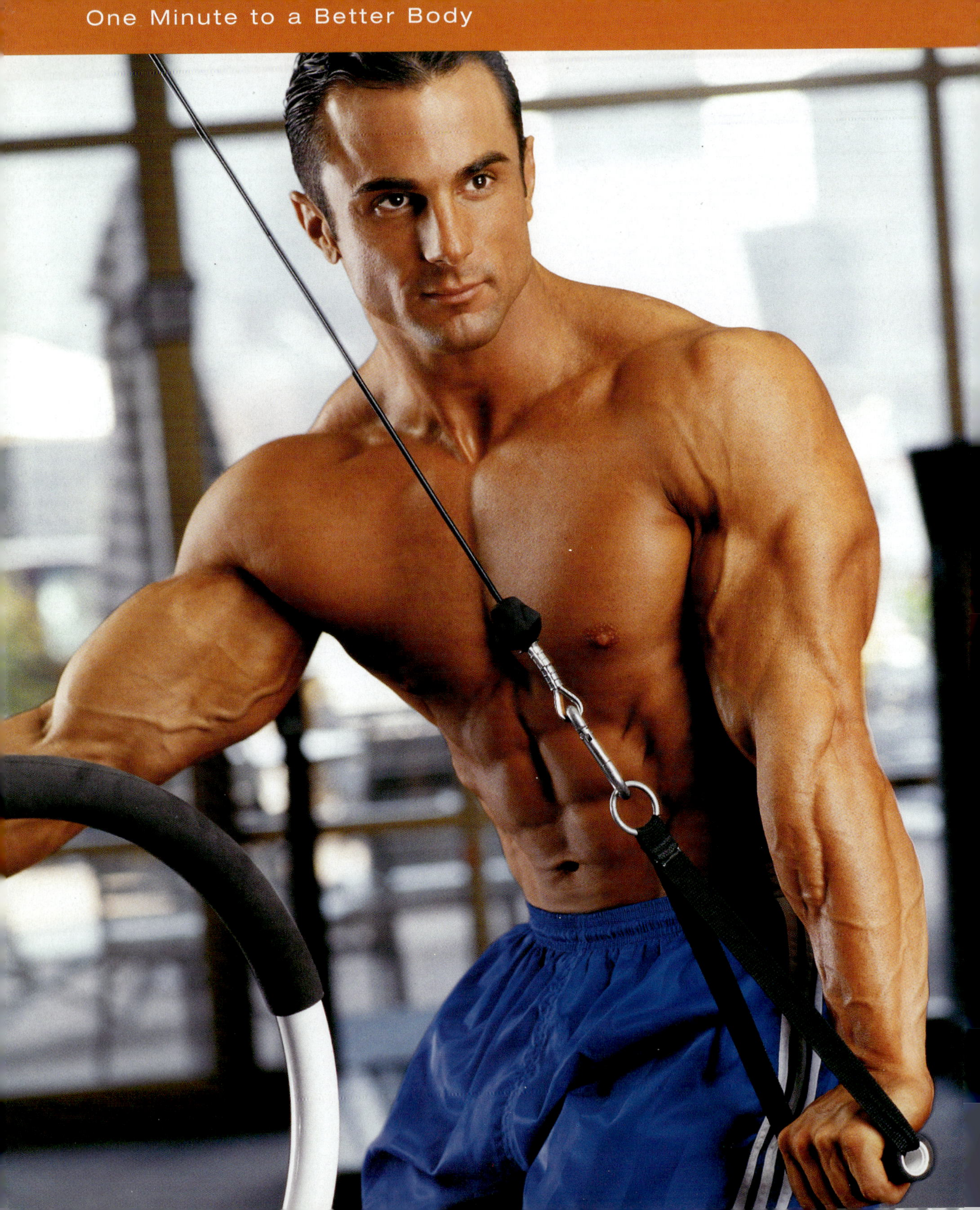

BASIC TRAINING

Understanding resistance training and what it can do for you

Anyone who's flipped through half a dozen muscle magazines can tell you a few things about resistance training. For instance, that if a person lifts weights regularly, that person is likely to increase muscle size and strength. And that a well-managed diet plays a huge role in this process as well. And maybe even that designing a workout program begins with having a clear idea of what one wants to achieve.

But take a good look at yourself in the mirror. You're someone who's committed to building a better body. And that means that you need to know a little more than that about the muscle-building process. Okay, a lot more. And if you're truly committed, you have to understand not only what works in the gym, but why.

It's toward that end that we've designed this section, to fill you in on some of the fundamental truths about resistance training. We'll cover all the basics, including the specific benefits of weightlifting, the science behind muscle growth, how to deal with soreness and injuries, and how to manipulate the "Triad of Success" to stay on track toward a fantastic physique.

Are you pumped? You should be — you're about to get your hands on the keys to total bodybuilding success. But, as you probably know, it's best to warm up before jumping into the heart of a work-

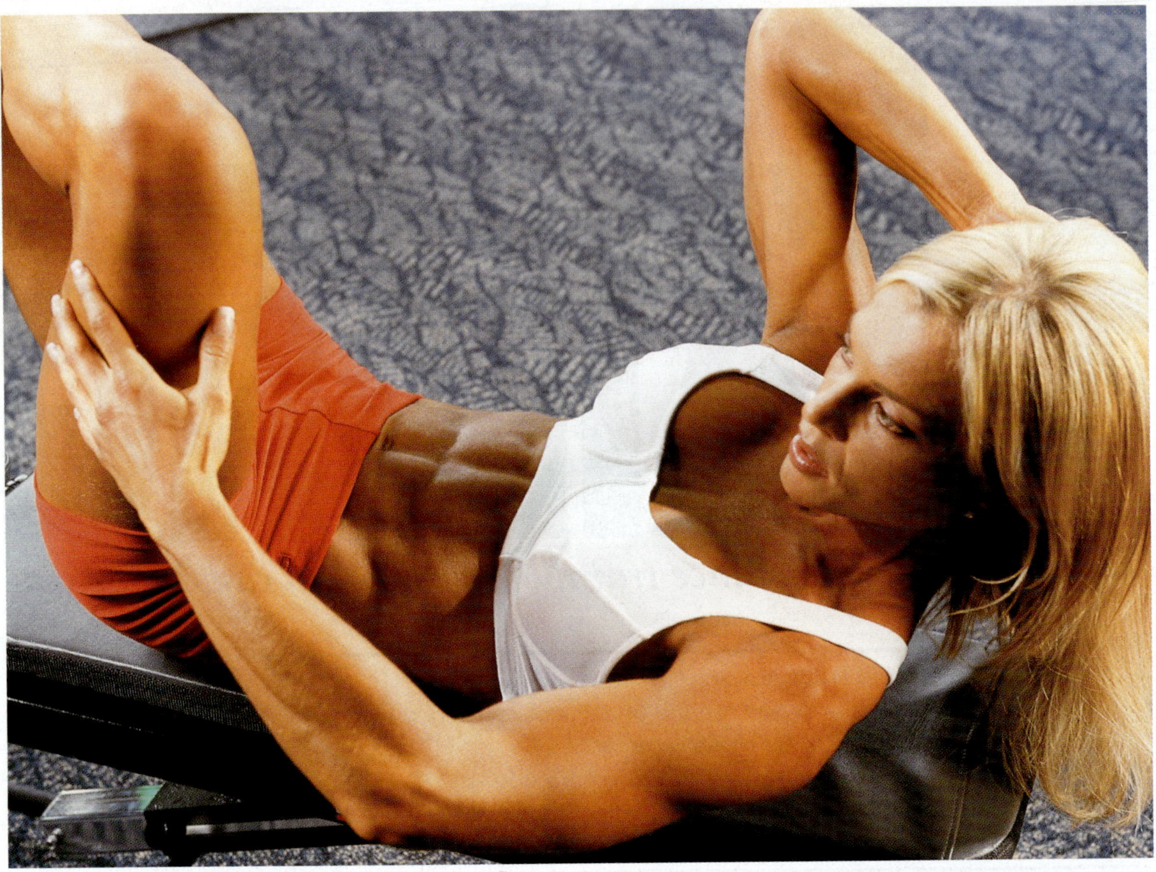

out. So, to warm your brain up for what you're about to learn, here are six Weider Principles, originally compiled by Joe Weider himself, that will give you a greater understanding of what works in resistance training, and, perhaps more important, why. Together with the one-minute lessons provided in this section, they're sure to make your next trip to the gym your best, most productive session yet.

Go for peak contraction. What: Hold the weight in the fully contracted position for a moment — up to two seconds — at the top of an exercise, concentrating on squeezing the muscle. Why: Holding a peak contraction intensifies the effort and counters the tendency of relaxing at the point of full contraction, when you've reached the end of the range of motion.

Use continuous tension. What: Maintain continuous tension on a given muscle throughout its entire range of motion. Why: To work a muscle fully, it needs to be stressed from its fully stretched position to one of peak contraction — its entire range of motion. Finding the right rep speed, minimizing momentum and working through the full range with proper form prevents injury and produces maximum development.

Confuse your muscles. What: Constantly change variables in your workout — number of sets, number of reps, exercise choice, length of your rest periods, etc.

Why: When your muscles become accustomed to a certain way of doing things, you're likely to hit a plateau, a point when your muscles grow slowly or not at all. Switching things up keeps you out of that rut by forcing your muscles to adapt and grow.

Perform multiple sets. What: Do more than one set for each exercise. Why: Performing multiple sets gives the target muscle a more thorough workout for optimal growth.

Split your bodyparts. What: Rather than doing a total-body routine, divide bodyparts over multiple workouts. For example, work chest and triceps one day, legs the next, shoulders and abs the third workout, and back and biceps on day four. Why: Following this principle will allow you to train individual bodyparts more completely and perform each workout with more intensity.

Finally, trust your instincts. What: Experiment and pay attention to the results of your training to help develop a feel for what works best for you. Why: When it comes to weight training, everybody is the same, yet everyone is different. The basics work for everyone, but the more advanced you get, the more you need to individualize your training cycles, intensity levels, reps, sets and diet. This isn't a random process; it takes a long time to discover what variations give you the best results, to develop a feel for how your body is responding. The more you're able to listen to your body and give it what it needs, the greater your progress will be.

That should be enough to kick-start your synapses. Now that you're revved up, keep reading. The best information, insight and knowledge are yet to come.

Basic Training: Questions and Answers

1
BIGGER AND BETTER

No question, resistance training builds an attractive physique, but what are some of the other health-related benefits that might help me as I grow older?

A: Exercise is widely recognized as the common denominator in the quest for good health. Resistance training specifically has several benefits: Not only does it figure heavily in bodyweight control, but it lessens the risk of a host of ills such as cardiovascular problems, diabetes, several types of cancer and more. In one test, researchers at Johns Hopkins University (Baltimore) found that the transit time of food

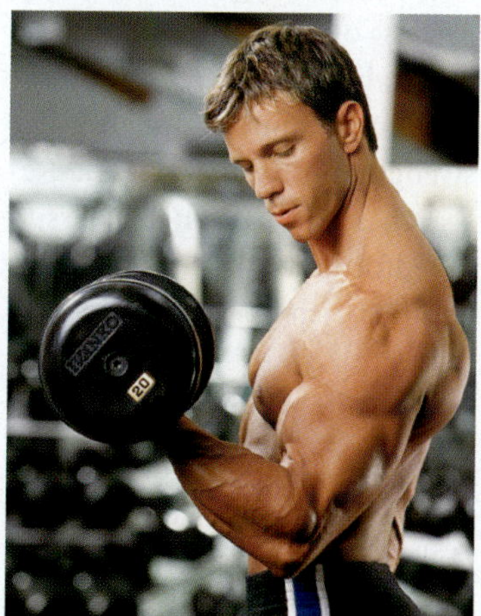
Weight training decreases the risk of cardiovascular problems and diabetes.

through the intestine was shortened by half after subjects engaged in three months of strength training, reducing the risk of such problems as diverticulitis, hemorrhoids, constipation and possibly colon cancer.

In addition, clinical trials have shown that resistance training reduces the "bad" LDL cholesterol while adding aerobic exercise raises the "good" HDL cholesterol. Talk about a one-two punch! This supports our belief that a combination of weight training and aerobics may be the ideal regimen for losing weight and improving cholesterol levels.

While a lifetime of fitness is the goal to strive for, many scientific studies in recent years show that lifting weights becomes increasingly important past age 50 in preventing such common causes of disability as brittle bones, back pain and instability. It can maintain or restore strength and vitality as well. Researchers at Tufts University (Medford, Massachusetts) also support the superiority of strength training for post-menopausal women: They found that while walking prevented bone loss only in the spine, resistance training actually thickened the bones of the spine and hips, reducing the chance for fractures in these vulnerable areas. This led to a greater capacity for overall activity that could help keep the bones strong.

The magic of progressive-resistance weight training is its fast-acting effect. For beginners, a single set of 8–12 repetitions per bodypart using a barbell, dumbbells, a machine or body-weight in a 20–30-minute full-body workout 2–3 times a week will start to build muscle, boost metabolism, fight low-back pain, increase bone density and shield the heart from overexertion. And it works for all ages and both genders.

2

REST ASSURED

I spend three hours each day in the gym, trying to work out seven days a week as I'm fairly small for my height. A guy told me that the muscles actually grow when I'm not in the gym, and that I'm not getting enough rest for this to occur. Is that right?

A: MUSCLE & FITNESS preaches that if you lift, eat and rest, the muscle will come. True, but the science behind it all runs deep. So much so that exercise scientists rack their brains for hours on end so that you can get bigger. We won't go to those lengths, but the more you know about what goes on under your skin, the more apt you'll be to pack on muscle. Here's how it works:

You Lift and Break Down Your Muscles

The continuous shortening (concentric) and lengthening (eccentric) of your muscles that occurs when you lift weights causes damage in the muscle tissue. Protein filaments called actin and myosin (found in the muscle fibers or cells) that cause your muscles to contract undergo microtrauma. This is actually microscopic tears in the fibers that cause the soreness you feel days after an intense lifting session. Don't worry, it isn't as bad as it sounds.

At Rest the Muscles Rebuild Themselves

In response to the damage that lifting has induced, your muscle fibers react by rebuilding themselves. But instead of simply growing back to where they were before, the fibers actually

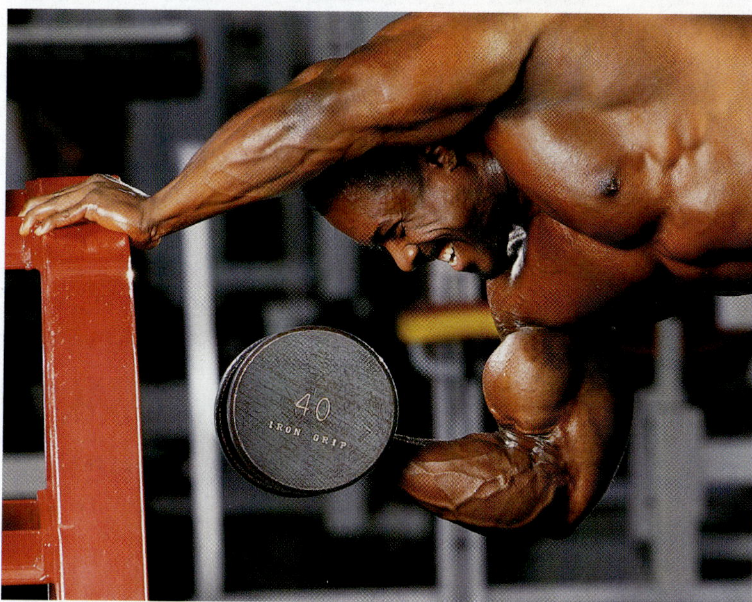

When you lift weights, muscle fibers tear. Rest allows them to rebuild.

produce more actin and myosin and, as a result, become bigger. This is referred to as hypertrophy. In a nutshell, this is how lifting weights creates larger muscles.

Without Adequate Rest Muscles Don't Rebuild

Inducing minor muscle tears is one thing; lifting excessively and not supplying your body with sufficient rest and the proper nutrients to support muscle building are another. Muscle fibers begin to repair themselves within minutes after damage occurs and the process can take several days. If you damage your muscles without giving them the rest they need – and that means getting enough sleep and not overly taxing yourself outside the gym – they won't have time to rebuild. When this doesn't happen, neither does hypertrophy. And that's why it isn't wise to train the same muscle group two days in a row.

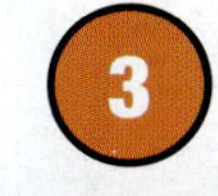

SORENESS & GROWTH

Some days I'm not sore after a workout, even though I trained

to failure or past failure. Will I see equal muscle growth after sessions when I'm sore and when I'm not? I constantly change my routines, always doing something different. Am I training hard enough? Should muscle soreness be a goal?

A: Muscle soreness should definitely not be your goal. The soreness you experience after a workout essentially comes about because you damaged your muscle fibers. Exercise physiologists refer to this as delayed-onset muscle soreness (DOMS), and it typically becomes most noticeable a day or two after a workout. What happens is that microtears in your muscle fibers cause calcium leakage via several mechanisms, causing you to experience an accumulation of histamines, potassium, prostaglandins and local edema in the affected muscle. The edema stimulates the nerve endings, causing the sensation of pain.

The damage to your muscles

and subsequent soreness occur to a greater degree during the negative (eccentric) component of an exercise. Possibly that's why you don't always experience the same level of soreness; not all exercises place the same type of eccentric stress on your muscles.

Now, you've probably ing to the stress of training, and you won't experience the same type of pain unless you increase the stress to an even greater degree. But I have to ask you: How much harder can you train? At some point, it would seem that you'd have to train till you fall over in each set. That's hardly reasonable.

extensive that you constantly experience DOMS. In fact, if you do, you're on the right track to becoming overtrained, in which case you can kiss your gains goodbye and say hello to an increased chance of injury.

The best way to go about your training is to manipulate

'The best way to go about your training is to manipulate how intensely you train over time, and do the same thing with your training volume and frequency.'

noticed that the amount of soreness decreases as you become more accustomed to a particular workout and/or exercise. You're basically adapt-

A certain amount of damage to muscles seems to be required for increases in strength and size to occur. But the damage need not be so

how intensely you train over time, and do the same thing with your training volume and frequency. Termed periodization, this has been found to be the most effective training system. The basic premise is that you'll observe times of highly intense training followed by less-intense training. A good textbook to check out is *Designing Resistance Training Programs* by Steven Fleck and William Kraemer (Human Kinetics, 1997).

A little bit of stiffness is probably to be expected after almost all workouts, but if you end up being sore for more than one day, you probably went too far. Make sure this doesn't happen too frequently.

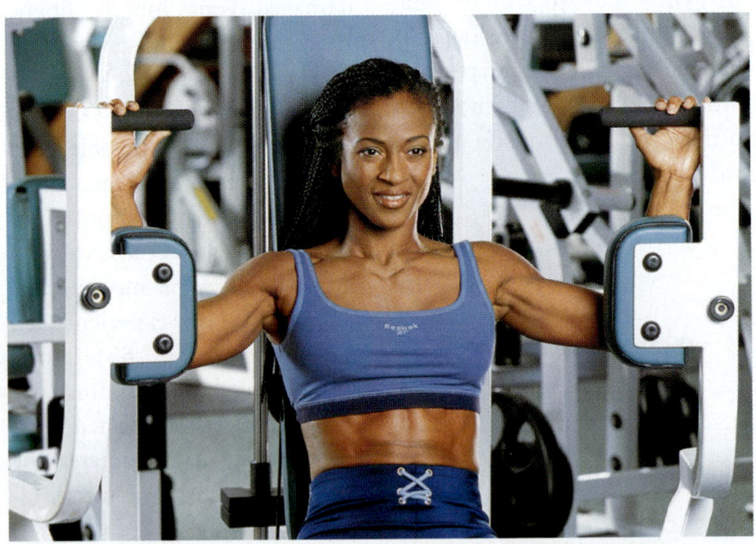

As your muscles adapt to the stress of training, soreness will decrease.

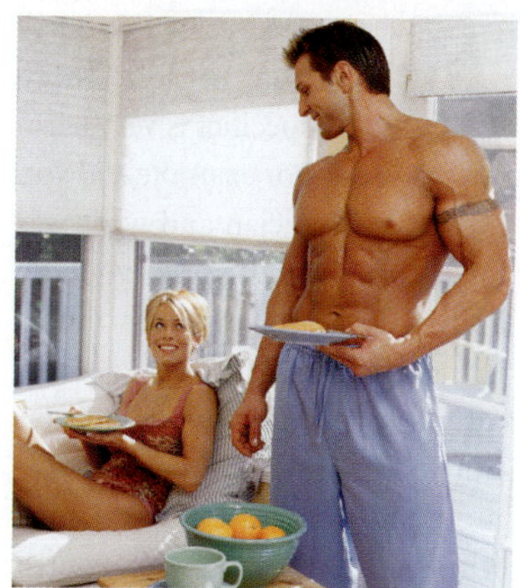

Eating nutrient-rich foods will help your muscles grow to their full potential.

THE TRIAD OF SUCCESS

I'm lifting hard but the gains are slow to non-existent. What can I do to get back on track?

A: All bodybuilders experience periods of slow or halted growth. Although frustrating, such plateaus are a normal part of training and must be accepted as such. They typically don't last long and can often be fixed with a slight change in your workout routine or by simply taking a few days off. Occasionally, the slump lingers for what seems like an eternity. When a few weeks of stale workouts becomes a few months, you know the time has come to take a serious look at your training regimen.

Of the many variables involved in a successful bodybuilding program, the time spent pumping iron is ordinarily deemed the most important. Although weight training is significant, other factors can be as crucial in the overall plan. When examining your routine for areas of needed improvement, focus on training first, but also look beyond the gym. Don't forget the critical roles that diet, rest and personal feedback play in muscle development.

Muscles cannot grow to their full potential without adequate nutrition. Supplements complement a balanced diet, but don't provide ample nutrition on their own (that's why they're called "supplements"). Eat a variety of unprocessed, nutrient-dense foods to ensure that your body gets the vitamins and minerals it needs to function properly. Consume sufficient calories in the proper ratio of carbs, protein and fat to provide your body

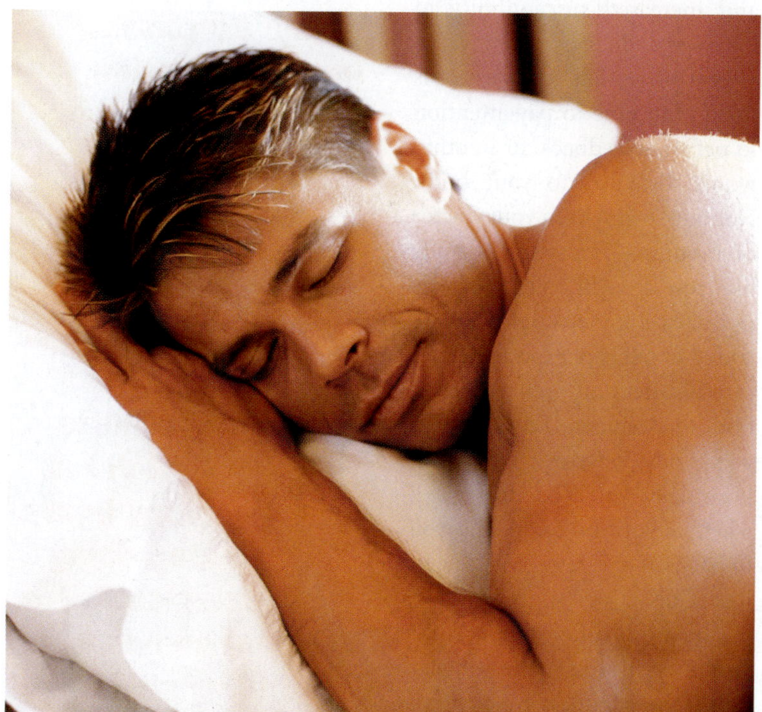

Rest is an important component of a successful bodybuilding program.

with the fuel it needs to train hard and build muscle.

Rest is the third component, together with training and diet, that forms the necessary basis for success. Contrary to what some people think, muscle growth occurs during rest, not while training. Training tears muscle tissue down (ironically, making the body weaker and more susceptible to infection). Ensuing rest, in the presence of nutrients, allows the body to recover and rebuild. Without sufficient rest, the body cannot fully recover, resulting in decreased strength and increased susceptibility to injury and illness.

Part of getting enough rest is taking the time to pay attention to personal feedback, or in other words, listening to your body. Nobody — not even your doctor or mother — knows your body like you do. Although you may not always understand what it's trying to tell you, experience and careful attention will teach you how to decipher the signs that your body constantly sends you. Eventually, you'll be able to tell whether your body's telling you to back off and rest, or if it's saying, "Go!"

The next time you feel like you're spinning your wheels, assess the situation by examining your training, diet and rest habits. Or better yet, keep these parameters in constant check, and maybe you can avoid training slumps altogether.

5

INJURY DILEMMA

For quite some time now, I've been rehabilitating a shoulder injury that I suffered while doing an incline bench press. I do the exercises (internal rotation, shoulder abduction, horizontal abduction, etc.) that my physical therapist instructed me to do, but my shoulder doesn't feel any stronger and sometimes it hurts worse than it did at the time of my injury. Should I stop doing these exercises? If so, what should I do to help my shoulder recover properly?

A: Answering this question without more specifics is very hard. For example, did you ever see a physician and what was his or her diagnosis? Do you still bodybuild? If so, at what volume, intensity and frequency? How often do you do your rehabilitation exercises and at what volume and intensity? Does it hurt while you do them or afterward? Are you taking any kind of medications (such as nonsteroidal anti-inflammatories)?

It's difficult to give you solid advice without more details, but you should keep some basics in mind. For one, don't do anything that hurts you. Train around the injury. If an exercise hurts, substitute it with one that doesn't. If this means that your delt/pec training ends up being next to nil, so be it. One thing we can promise you: If you continue to push it, not only will it get worse but you may create a chronic problem that you'll have to deal with for the rest of your life.

Richard T. Herrick, MD, an accomplished masters powerlifter and weightlifter, is also the chief medical officer for the International Powerlifting Federation and the United States Weightlifting Federation. He agrees that we don't have enough

'If you continue to push it, you may create a chronic problem that you'll have to deal with for the rest of your life.'

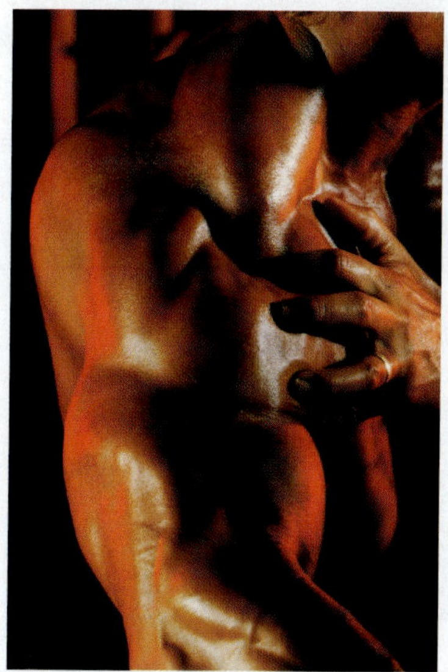

Always train around an injury, avoiding movements that cause any pain.

information for an accurate diagnosis, but he suspects you may have either an impingement, rotator-cuff tear or A/C joint sprain (the acromioclavicular joint is toward the tip of your collarbone). By all means, have a physician check you out or re-evaluate the injury. This should include a physical exam to determine any areas of weakness and/or pain. If this exam doesn't provide sufficient answers, it may be time to get X-rays or an MRI, or to utilize other diagnostic tools. As a final caveat, Herrick believes the rehabilitation exercises you've been doing may not be sufficient. Talk to your physician or athletic trainer about various stretching movements you could employ, how to do them correctly and at what frequency. ∎

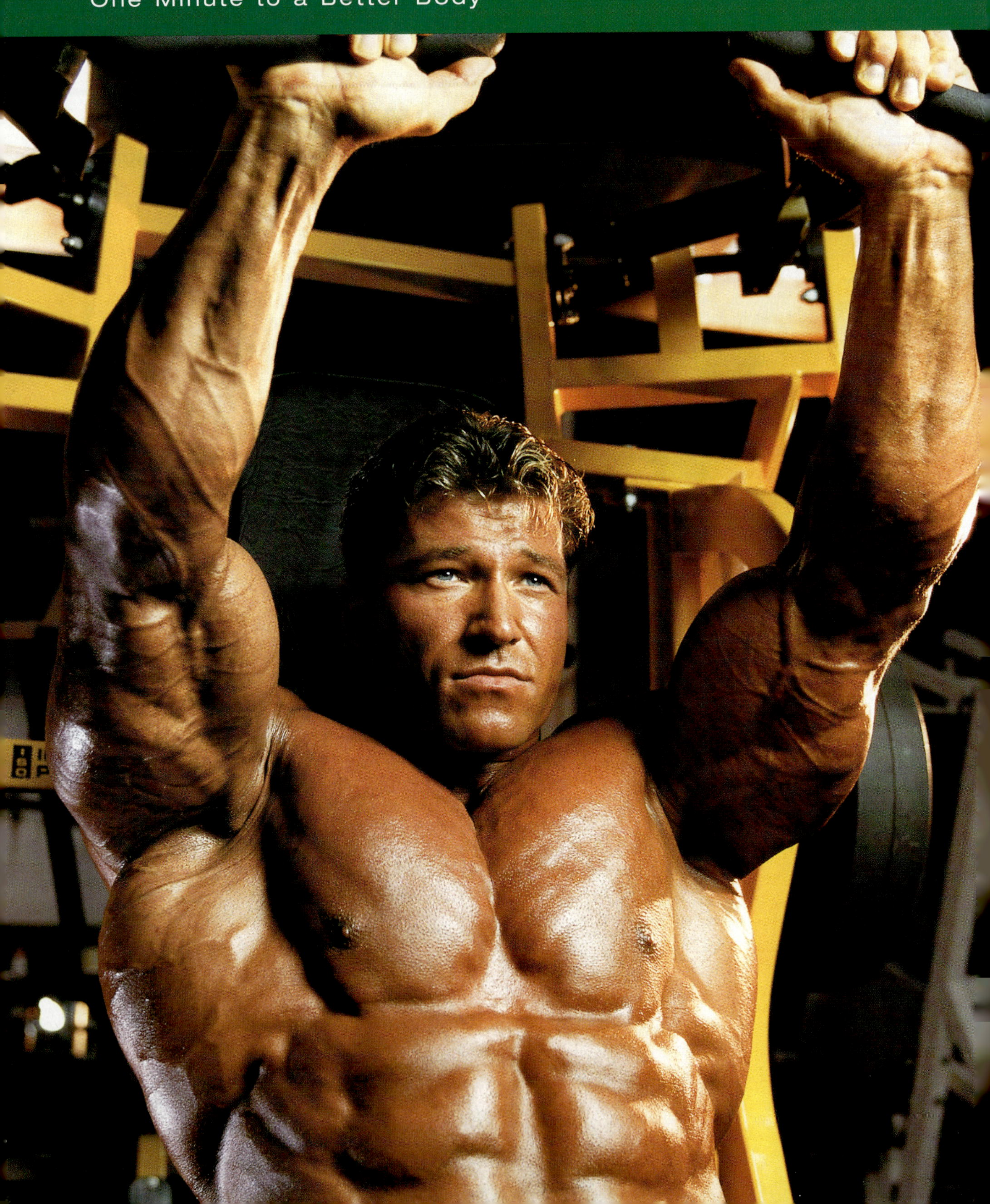

ELEMENTS OF YOUR WORKOUT

Fine-tuning the variables that make up your routine

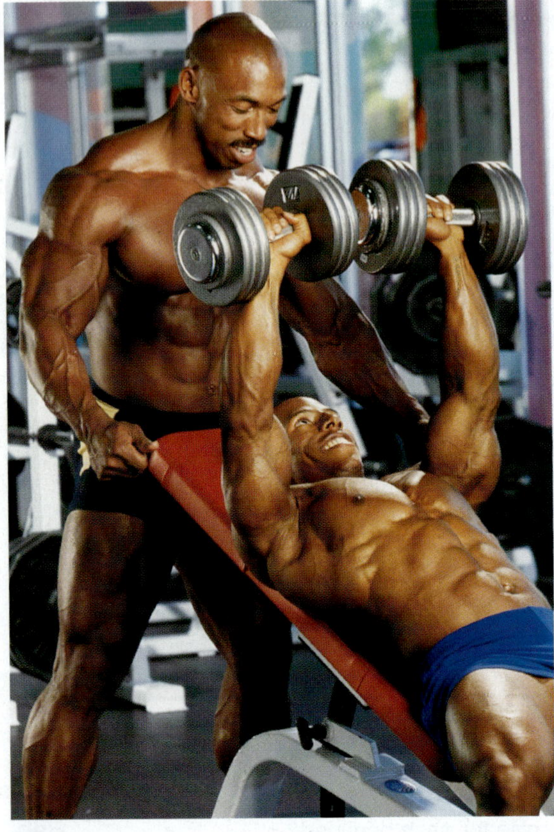

I t's the nature of human physiology: Training progress can come in trickles, in a steady stream or not at all. Unfortunately, you often don't realize you've reached a plateau until you've been stuck on one too long. Maybe you haven't made strength gains, added muscle or dropped bodyfat. At this point in the game, you can take one of two roads: 1) Hit the gym and do what you've been doing all along, but harder and more often, or 2) Regard your plateau as a signal to change. Obviously, the latter is the way to go, but most of us persist with the former. To avoid the worst-case scenario, where motivation wanes, workouts are skipped and gains slip away, heed the following advice.

Start by assessing your goals. Are you looking to shed 20 pounds of fat or add 15 pounds of muscle? Hiring a certified personal trainer — even for a few sessions — can save you time, money and frustration in the long run. Find an accredited professional, articulate your goals and ask for a six-week road map. Aim to achieve muscle development, good flexibility and overall coordination. Consider the time you have to devote to exercise and be realistic.

Split your workouts. A suitable program for a beginner (typically someone in his or her first year of training) consists of three full-body workouts a week, separated by recovery days. Intermediate-level trainees might want to separate push-pull upper-body muscle groups over those three days, working chest, shoulders and triceps on day 1, legs and calves on day 2, and back and biceps on day 3.

Even if you already split your workout, try new pairings to break up your old routine. If you always train arms after a larger bodypart, you'll be surprised at how much you can push them when you do an arms-only training day.

Kick up the intensity level. You can rev up your intensity by either adding some reps (be it forced reps in which a workout partner helps you push past your sticking point to complete additional reps, or partial reps in which you do a few extra reps at the end of your set through a very short range of motion, etc.)

'Start by assessing your goals. Are you looking to shed 20 pounds of fat or add 15 pounds of muscle?'

to each set. This means extending a set past the point where it normally ends because of muscular failure. Don't be afraid to use advanced training techniques on occasion (assuming you're an advanced intermediate), but don't do them on all sets, and make sure you're well rested before you start your next set. Maintain energy by cycling high-intensity workouts with moderate-intensity workouts for recovery.

Educate yourself on the newest and latest. Read books on exercise (like this one) or study exercise descriptions in MUSCLE & FITNESS, being on the lookout for new ways to do old favorites. Learn about proper body alignment and controlling your torso and limbs through the movement. Train yourself to utter key phrases before each exercise: feet planted, knees bent, abs tight, chest lifted, shoulders back, etc. Advanced trainees automatically incorporate a quick

"body check," putting themselves into proper lifting posture before they begin a movement.

Increase your arsenal of exercises. There are more than 20 exercises for each bodypart, so why should you stick with the same 3-4 over and over again? Learn new movements, practice them and use them in your workout. Remember, though, not all exercises substitute equally for one another. You won't want to switch over to a steady diet of cable crossovers in place of your heavy benches, or leg extensions instead of squats. Make compound exercises the backbone of your workout, and train in the rep range that delivers mass-building results. No matter what level you're at, keep your ego out of it, focusing on technique and movement. Beginners should keep the weight light as you learn the movement (stay between 12-15 reps). Don't dip

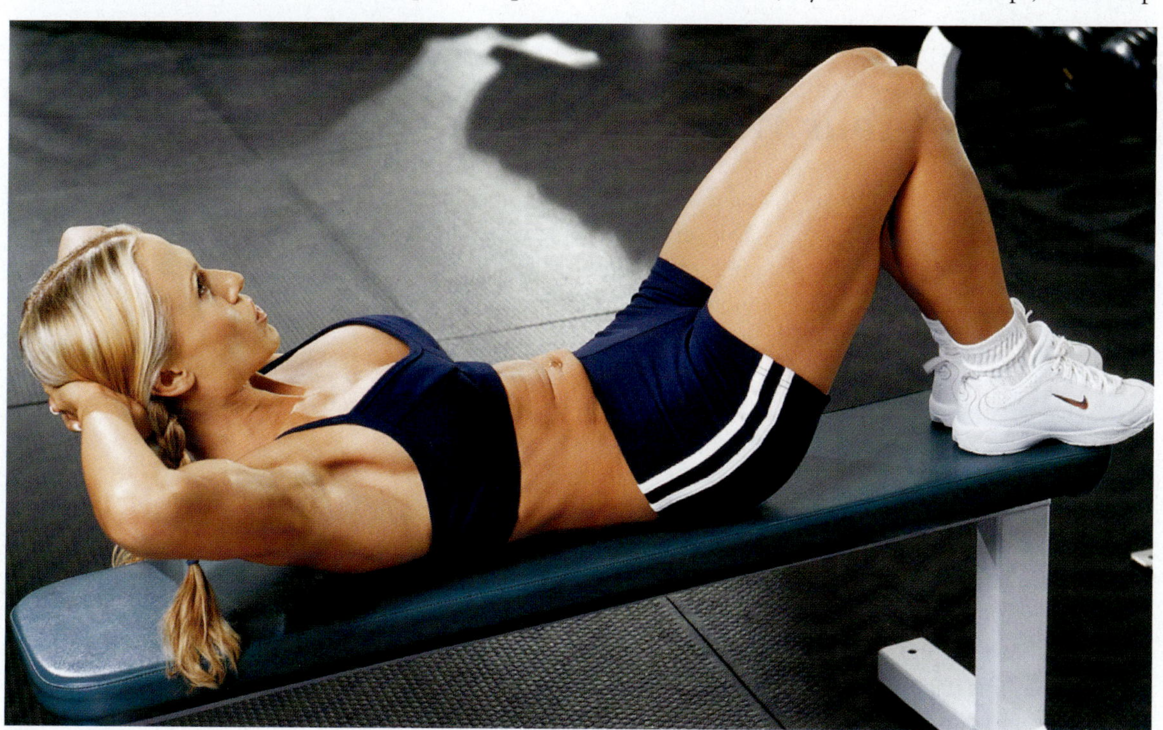

lower than six reps in a set, which gets into powerlifter territory; you'll maximize strength using this weight.

Use single-joint isolation exercises to complement your compound movements. Single-joint exercises like lying leg curls and leg extensions employ a single-joint action while isolating the target muscle. Compound (or multijoint) exercises are somewhat more difficult, entailing movement through at least two joints, and require greater neuromuscular control. With multijoint movements forming the basis of your routine, add single-joint exercises to finish off the working muscle. You can usually go a little lighter for higher reps here, focusing on really building a muscle burn.

Find a training partner to push you. You can also do a number of advanced training techniques with a partner, extending a set well past the point where you'd normally quit. Push each other in a friendly but competitive way.

Try advanced exercises. Many movements, like Olympic lifts, walking lunges and one-legged squats, require total-body strength and coordination. Incorporate a few of them, starting with very light weights to get the hang of the movement. Get a trainer to guide and spot you with tricky exercises. You might want to incorporate some elements of a pro bodybuilder's routine, but watch the number of sets and leave the reps on the high end.

Read on for more tips on building your workout routine. From using free weights to the optimal number of sets, this section covers every part of your muscle-building routine.

Elements of Your Workout: Questions and Answers

MUSCLE PREP

What's the best way to warm up before starting a workout, and is stretching an effective means?

A: The purpose of "warming up," as the expression implies, is to increase blood flow to your muscles and raise your core body temperature. This effectively increases joint mobility and makes muscles more elastic. Common sense also suggests that warm muscles are less susceptible to injury, although research isn't conclusive in support of this theory.

While stretching in itself can warm up muscle tissue and loosen joints, it should never be used as your primary warm-up activity. In fact, the benefits of stretching are best realized when it's done after a complete warm-up that includes moderate, low-

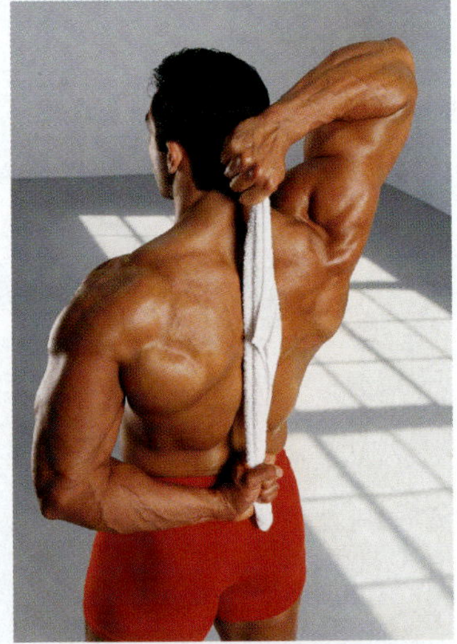
Stretch only after a cardio warm-up.

impact aerobic activity. The aerobic activity you select to kick off your warm-up routine should involve a repetitive, low-impact movement that utilizes the larger muscle groups for 5–10 minutes. Any activity that raises your heart rate and elevates your core body temperature is good, but rowing machines and some cross-training machines are particularly useful because they involve your legs and back (as well as the chest, in the case of the latter). As soon as you start to break a sweat, your muscles should be sufficiently warmed up and ready for more vigorous activity.

After 10 minutes of cardio warm-up, it's safe to stretch your muscles. Although some research suggests that stretching warms the deep muscle fibers, little evidence supports the immediate benefits of stretching before lifting weights for bodybuilders and other athletes. For this reason, many lifters choose to stretch after their workouts, when their muscles are the warmest and most pliable. Under these conditions, the best results are achieved when stretches are held for at least 30 seconds.

Following your general warm-up, make sure you go through a specific warm-up before you begin high-intensity training.

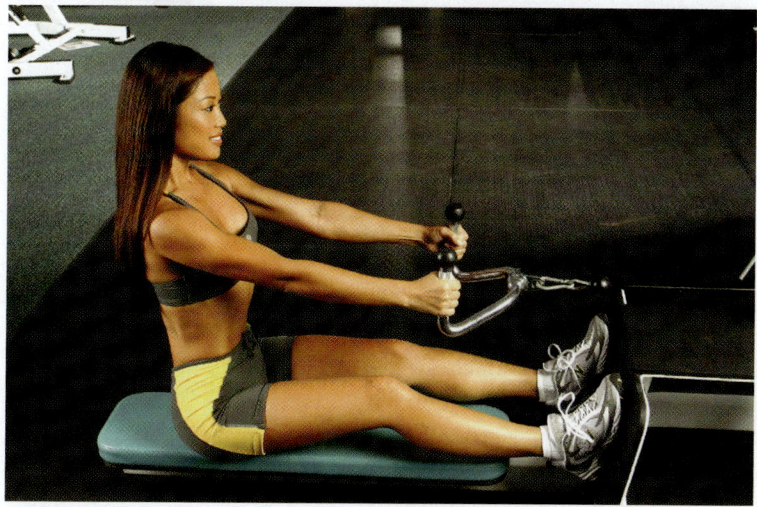
Machines are a safe alternative to free weights for a beginning bodybuilder.

Start each exercise with several light warm-up sets to get the muscles, joints and mind ready for the work to come. Whether you stretch before hitting the iron is your personal choice. Just remember, always start with 5–10 minutes of cardio to warm up before your warm-up.

7

SET YOURSELF FREE

I'm fairly new to weight training. I was taught a number of basic movements on machines, but have heard that using free weights is superior for muscle building. In fact, it's even intimidating to go in there, as everyone seems to know what they're doing, except me. Should I stick to free weights or can I get comparable results with machines?

A: Many people shun free weights — called barbells and dumbbells — out of such intimidation. Using machines can also be safer and easier, especially at first. But if you

29

want the most for your efforts, don't be afraid to head straight toward the free-weight room.

Why Free Weights?

Free weights offer a number of physiological benefits that machines cannot. Foremost, training with free weights recruits more muscle fibers than using machines. Machines isolate muscle groups so they build strength in a specific area. For example, a chest-press machine will build strength only in the area of the pec muscle targeted by that machine. On the other hand, if you used free weights to do the same movement, you would build strength in more than one area. Because you're hitting many other muscle groups, you'll end up working a larger part of your body.

Moreover, while machines limit movement to only one plane of motion, the varied movements used with free weights mimic the way we move naturally. In everyday life you don't move in merely one direction. Free weights more closely mimic the way you move naturally and when playing sports. So they not only work more of your muscles than machines, but also build strength that will help you outside the gym.

8

ARRESTED DEVELOPMENT

I work out regularly, but I can't seem to get definition in my calves and biceps. What exercises do you recommend for these muscle groups?

A: People commonly ask questions like this. Most of the time it's because they aren't seeing the development they want in a particular bodypart and they believe a bet-

ter exercise is out there.

Herein lies the problem. The reality is that some of us won't develop as much as others, and we all tend to have bodyparts that just don't want to respond to training. What this means is that no matter what you do, that lagging bodypart probably won't magically turn into one of your best.

Now, don't get us wrong — We're not suggesting that you just give up on your bi's if they're weaker than your tri's. By all means, seek out ways to trick those suckers into growing. But at the same time, understand that your genetics play a large part here; you might be somewhat limited in this particular bodypart. And if you look around, you'll see that you aren't alone.

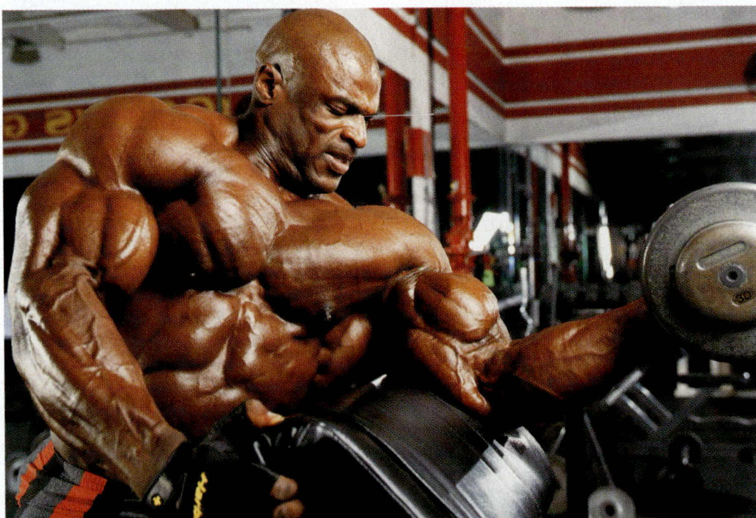

Genetics play a role in how much muscle groups, like the biceps, will grow.

Bill Grant had weak calves, as did Roy Callender. Chris Dickerson came in short in the biceps department, and Boyer Coe likely did everything short of transplantation surgery to get a six-pack. Nevertheless, each one became a champion bodybuilder.

This also means that you probably have many bodyparts that respond well to training and have excellent development. Maybe you're one of those people who can, for example, put an inch on your quads by just looking at a squat rack. Why is that? Genetics! Bottom line, there's no such thing as a best exercise for any given bodypart. Essentially, your exercise selection ends up being a choice between multijoint and single-joint movements. Multijoint exercises will give you more bang for your buck because, as in the bench press, your delts and tri's contribute as you emphasize your chest. On the other hand, a single-joint exercise such as the pec-deck flye will target just your pecs.

Does this mean one group of exercises is better than the other? If your goal is to maximize your growth, no. Do a range of exercises and use a variety of set, rep and intensity schemes. Allow ample time, about 4–5 weeks, for changes to occur. If you don't notice any appreciable changes,

realize that Mother Nature may be the limiting factor and move on to the next routine. Keep training and enjoy the process, like getting a pump. Just because you can't see growth doesn't mean you aren't getting something out of your workouts.

KEYS TO GROWTH

In an attempt to build size and strength, are the bench press, deadlift and squat adequate for a bodybuilding routine? If so, how regularly should I do them and where should they fit into the overall scheme of my program? Do sets, reps and intensity change in these exercises over others?

A: In answering your question, two main factors need to be considered: your training status and your goals.

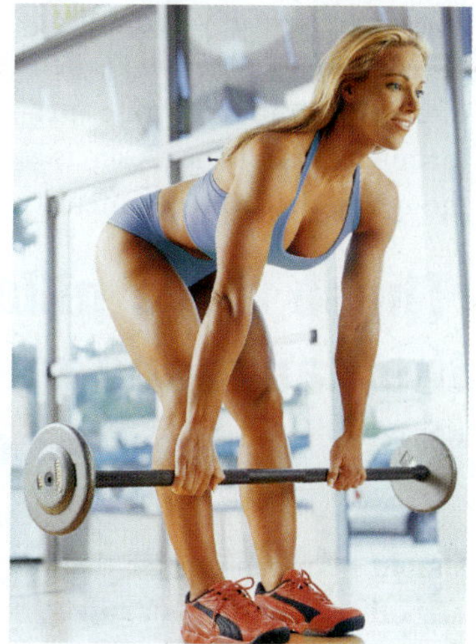

You'll get more gains from the deadlift than a single-joint movement.

The former is in reference to your level of experience in pumping iron. If you're a rank beginner, you might want to hold off on these exercises until you master some easier ones first. Good choices would be single-joint movements, because you can learn how to do them more easily and begin growing more quickly.

Now, if you have about 4–6 months of training experience and you're knocking on the intermediate bodybuilders' door, it's time to start doing the squat, bench and deadlift. Because these exercises are more difficult to learn and require more muscles to perform them, the long-term gains in strength and size will be greater than with single-joint exercises. If you're an advanced bodybuilder, you definitely want to continue performing these major exercises, though your level of intensity

Though you could do just squats on leg day, you'll get bored with that and will also compromise your gains. The human body adapts specifically to the exercis-

On chest day, for example, start with about four sets of benches and follow that up with dumbbell and cable work. For legs, start with the squat and

'These three pillars of power must constitute the backbone of your program. This means including them at least once a week.'

should be much greater than at any other point in your career.

Because you want more size and strength, these three pillars of power must constitute the backbone of your program. This means including them at least once a week, but it doesn't mean this is all you need to do.

es you do, so if you were to only squat, your body would develop in only that dimension. Granted, the squat, press and deadlift have a rather large "dimension," but for overall conditioning, strength and size, you should train each bodypart with many different exercises.

move on to lunges and leg presses. On back day you could start with the deadlift, then do back extensions or another type of pulling movement (hang pull, high pull) and a few variations of rows and/or pull-downs or pull-ups.

Approach your sets, reps and intensity (how much weight you move) the same way for each exercise. If your training calls for five sets of five reps per exercise at a heavy intensity, do that for all your exercises. Maintain this level of work for about three weeks, then drop down to light work, where you might choose to skip the big three. This won't stall your gains; in fact, it will make you grow since you're allowing for more recuperation, and it will certainly give you a break from the monotony of performing the same exercises too frequently.

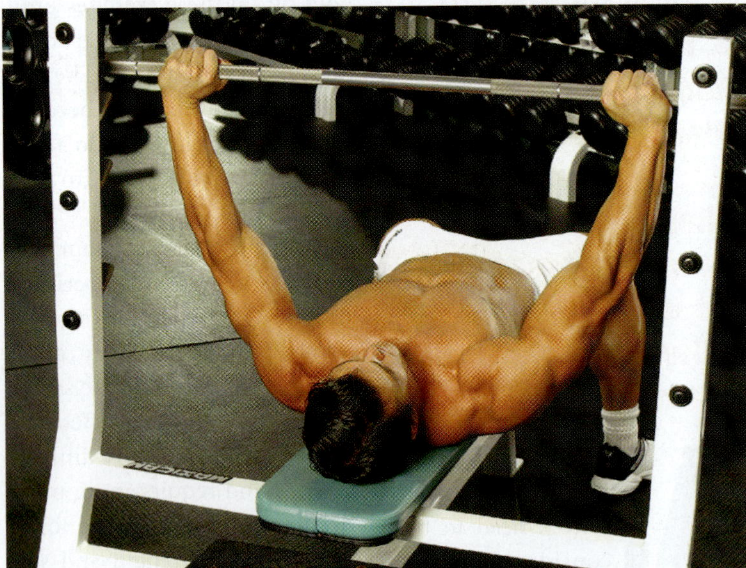

A bench press should be the backbone of your chest workout, not the only exercise.

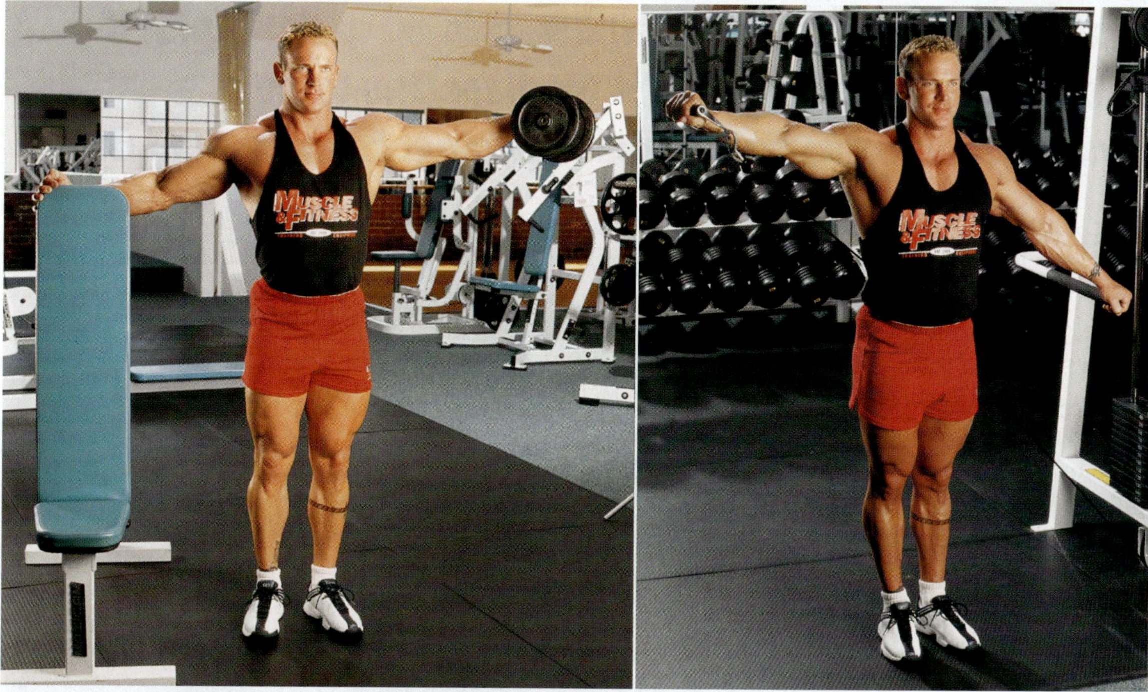

With dumbbells, the relative resistance changes throughout the movement. Cables provide constant tension but limit your angle of pull.

(10)

DUMBBELLS VS. CABLES

A: Resistance is resistance, right? You'd certainly think so, but it's true that the resistance can be slightly different to the working muscle, depending on the source. Deciding whether to use dumbbells or cables is partly a matter of preference, but also depends on your training goals. You need a brief review of physics to understand why 40 pounds of dumbbell resistance may not be quite the same as 40 pounds done on cables.

Let's say you're doing biceps curls with a 40-pound dumbbell. Although the absolute resistance remains constant at 40 pounds, the relative resistance (what your biceps feels) changes throughout the movement. From the bottom position of the curl, the relative resistance increases as you curl the dumbbell up, and it reaches maximum when your forearm is parallel to the floor. From here, the relative resistance decreases as the elbow-joint angle gets smaller and the dumbbell approaches your shoulder. That's why the weight seems heavier at the sticking

'The resistance of a dumbbell depends on gravity, with the force always directed toward the floor. The force of a cable, however, can come from directions other than straight down.'

point (forearm parallel to the floor) and lighter at the top of the movement.

The same principles hold true for cable movements, but the difference lies in the angle of resistance. The resistance of a dumbbell depends on gravity, with the force always directed toward the floor. The force of a cable, however, can come from directions other than straight down. Relative cable resistance also changes with elbow-joint position, but the changes are less dramatic with the appropriate cable angle. The most efficient angle is the one that follows the movement of the exercise as closely as possible, resulting in more consistent and continuous tension — the leading benefit of cable movements.

To help you better grasp this concept, visualize performing one-arm lateral raises with a cable. Typically you'd stand about 1–3 feet from the weight stack, depending on your height; that's the most comfortable position because of the cable angle. To complete the lateral raise, you abduct your arm up from your side until it's about parallel to the floor. This angular movement completes 90 degrees of a full circle. If you drew a

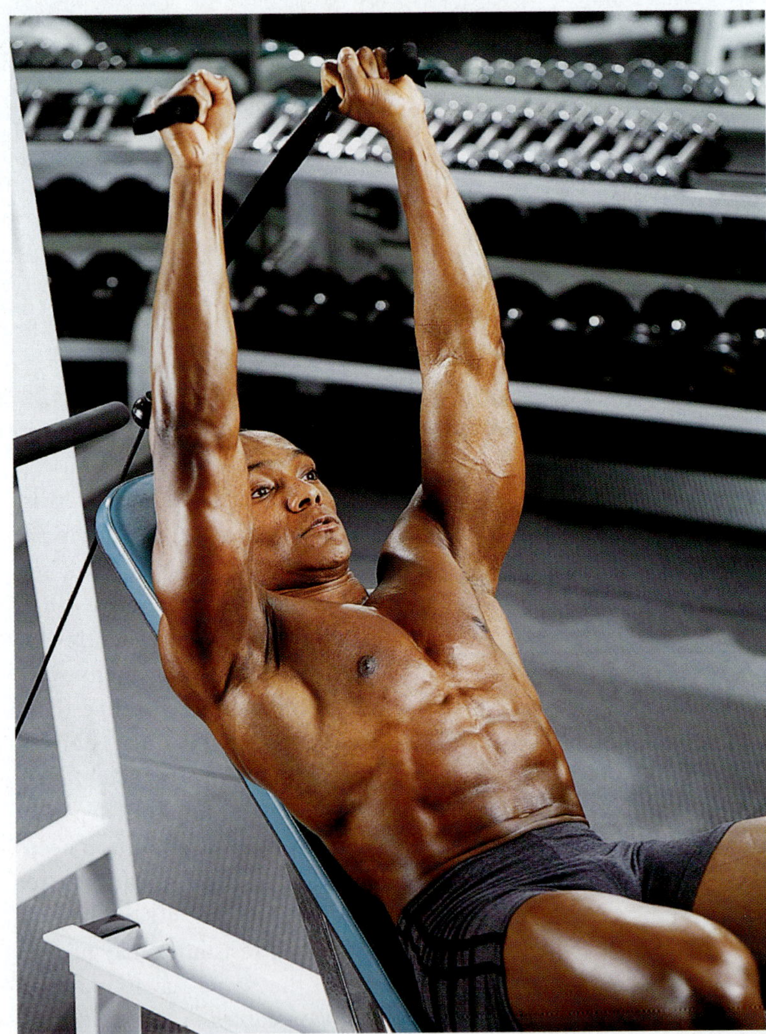

For best results, aim for a cable angle that follows the movement of the exercise.

straight line from your hand's position at the start of the movement to your hand's position at the top of the movement, it would make a 45-degree angle from the floor. By standing 1–3 feet away from the weight stack, you position the cable angle close to 45 degrees, which closely follows the movement of your hand during the lateral raise. If you stand closer to the stack, you decrease the cable angle (in relation to the vertical weight stack); if you move farther away, you increase it. While a cable angle smaller or larger than 45 degrees will cause greater variations in tension during the movement, at 45 degrees you'll find the "groove," and you should notice more consistent and continuous tension.

The potential drawback of cable movements is that the cable directs and limits the angle of pull to a certain extent. Doing so utilizes fewer assistant and stabilizer muscles, which are important for overall strength and development. On the flip side, decreased assistant/stabilizer involvement leads to greater stress of the target muscle. Both are desirable training tools, depending on your training focus. Maybe the drawback of cable movements isn't really a drawback after all.

So which type of resistance will ultimately lead to the development of more muscle and size — dumbbells or cables? The answer is "both;" variety is one of the most critical ingredients to a successful bodybuilding program. Variety is achieved through constantly exposing your muscles to different stimuli, including working them from different angles. Even though dumbbells and cables each have their own advantages, the benefits aren't significant enough to warrant exclusive use of either type of movement.

11

BODYWEIGHT BLUNDERS

On days that I'm not able to get to the gym, I'll do pull-ups, dips and push-ups. What's the sufficient number of reps and sets for these exercises, and how often should I do them? Do they promote muscle growth and strength?

A: Here's the bottom line: If you train about four days a week with weights, you don't need to do bodyweight exercises on your "off" days. In fact, in terms of your volume of work (how many sets and reps you do), more is worse when it comes to bodybuilding. Intensity (how hard you work or how much weight you lift), on the other hand, is a different story.

Assuming that with gym workouts and bodyweight exercises you train no more than five days a week, let's look at the relative value of pull-ups, dips and push-ups. If your goal is to get bigger and stronger, doing 15 reps or more with bodyweight only won't really help. It won't build a significant amount of muscle and, as for strength, you're actually just building endurance. Basically, the exercise lacks sufficient intensity.

To increase intensity and get enough of a growth stimulus, add weight to these exercises. Now we're talking about some of the most effective exercises you can do, period. With pull-ups, for example, start slowly by adding enough plates to a belt or strap so that you must decrease your reps to about 10 per set. Progressively add weight over time, but be sure to do at least five reps.

Try to push the intensity for no more than four weeks, then drop both weight and reps by 20%–30%; maintain the same number of sets per exercise and bodypart if you like. This allows your body to recover from all the hard work and you'll be stronger once you hit it heavy again. Try to find the ideal balance for hard training and recuperation weeks, and repeat that cycle for maximal gains.

12

SET SECRETS

Can you recommend an optimal number of sets per muscle group? I lift three times a week, hitting each muscle group hard at least one day with 8–9 sets, then lightly on a second day for 2–3 sets. My sets vary from 6–12 reps, depending on the muscle group and the amount of weight (fewer reps for heavier weights, typically on larger muscle groups). Could I be doing too many sets or too few sets?

A: You probably want a quick answer, preferably just a number, but unfortunately things aren't that easy. Ask any group of bodybuilders the same question and you'd get a different answer from each. A review of the research also gleans a variety of answers that depend on experience level, muscle group trained, type of exercise, exercise modality (such as dynamic or variable resistance), intensity, etc. As you can see, answering your question is a lot more complex than you might have thought.

What does seem clear from the research is that a beginner can make significant improvements in strength and body composition (building muscle and losing fat) by doing as little as one set per muscle group only two times a week. Of course, you don't remain a beginner forever, and you need to find ways to optimize your gains. To do that, research has clearly demonstrated that doing more than one set per muscle group or exercise is superior. Here, the optimal number seems to lie anywhere between five and 10.

Another training variable — intensity, or the amount of weight you lift — is more important than the actual number of sets you do. Research has shown that those who lift progressively heavier weights make better gains in strength and size

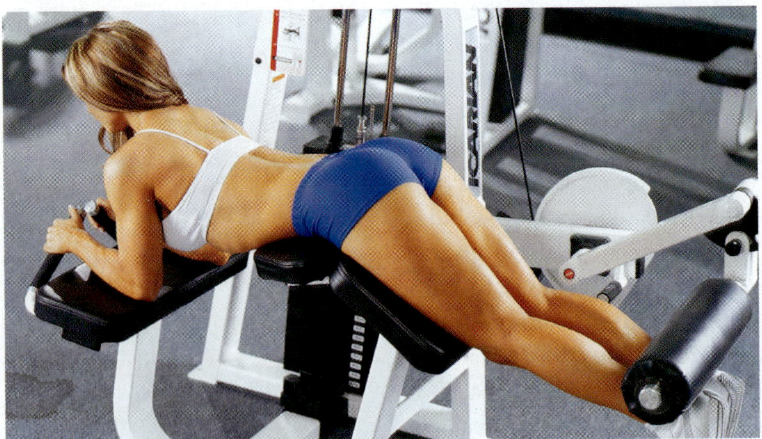

Utilize periodization during your training by varying your sets, reps and weight.

over those who vary only the number of sets. The best way to approach this is with a varying set, rep and weight scheme. This form of training is termed periodization, where you'd break a longer training period (several months) into smaller compo-

'Intensity, or the amount of weight you lift — is more important than the actual number of sets you do.'

nents (one to several weeks) and manipulate the sets, reps and intensity of your work in each component.

The number of sets you've selected seems fine. If you vary this number in relation to the amount of weight you use in each exercise, you'll be sure to maintain a growth spurt. Also consider frequency: You currently hit each muscle group twice a week, yet your best bet is to train only your arms and legs more than once a week. Try working your back, chest and shoulders with major exercises like the deadlift, power clean, high pull, etc., just once weekly.[1,2,3,4]

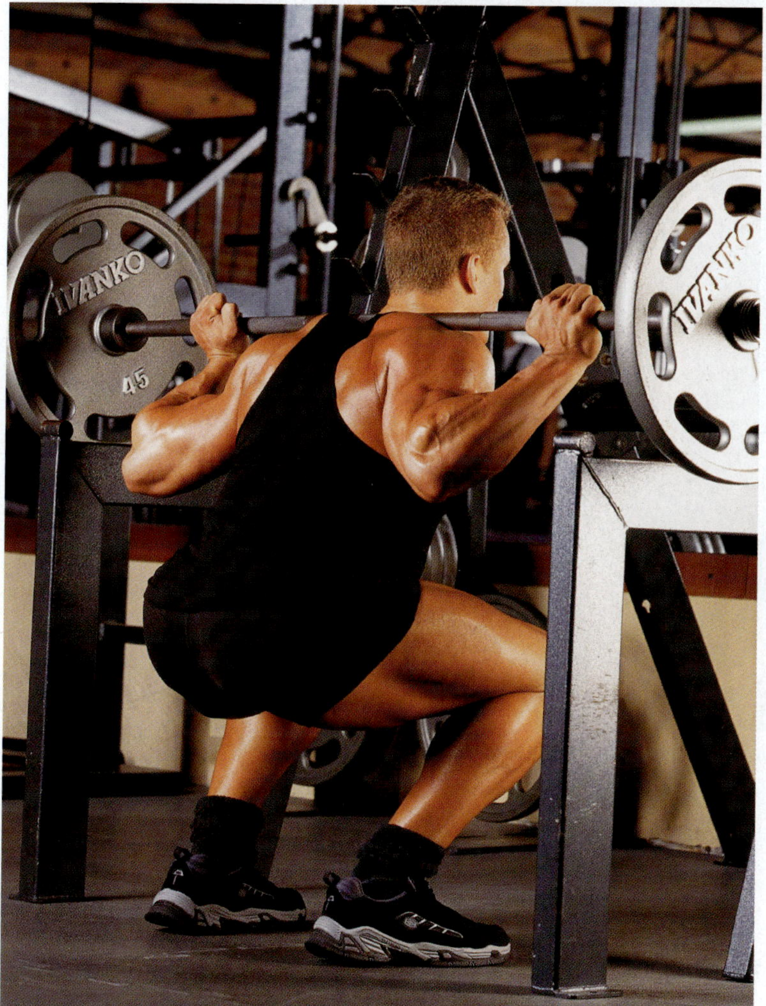

You should perform multiple sets of each exercise to optimize your gains.

13

ONE SET TO FAILURE

Is it possible for one set per exercise per session to be effective?

A: The issue of doing one set to failure can be viewed a few different ways. The

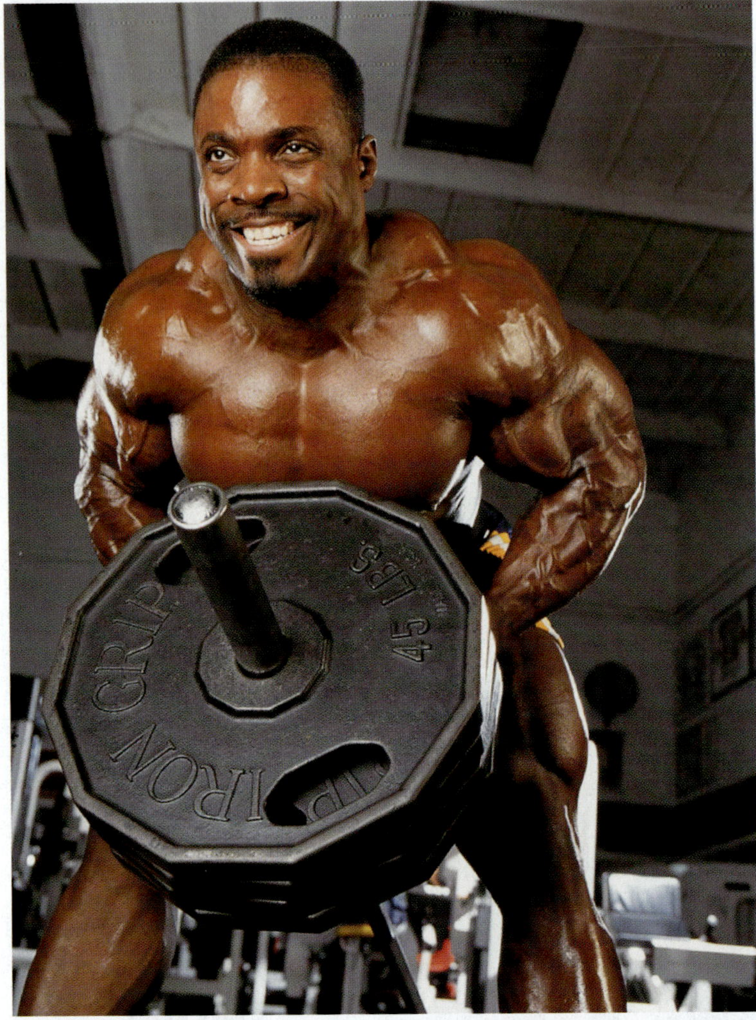

Performing one set to failure will not significantly improve your body composition.

American College of Sports Medicine considers training in this manner to be effective in terms of attaining general health. But let's assume you're a healthy and active person who wants to reach his or her potential in terms of physical development.

Conditioning should be an important training considera-tion. Bodybuilding isn't just about developing bigger mus-cles, it's also about condition-ing your body, raising it to the next level, so to speak. With that in mind, bigger muscles are just one part of the equa-tion. Don't forget about well-conditioned muscles that can perform repetitively without tiring. And what about body composition? How can you improve your body composi-tion to any significant degree if you perform only one set to failure? You simply won't expend enough calories to burn enough fat. So, if you do one set — even to failure — you'll condition yourself to only that level.

But let's take it one step further. When we talk about bodybuilding, we're really talk-ing about our bodies undergo-ing positive adaptations at many levels. Changes take place at a muscle-fiber level, connective tissues become stronger, your nervous system becomes more functional, cardiovascular changes occur, energy utilization becomes more efficient, your

'Bodybuilding isn't just about developing bigger muscles, it's also about conditioning your body.'

bones grow stronger and various hormonal adaptations take place as well.

Now, presumably, you'd like to know what research has to say on the subject of one set to failure. The truth is, not much. In one study conducted by B.F. Hurley and reported in the October 1984 issue of Medicine & Science in Sports & Exercise, researchers found that although the single-set paradigm offered significant increases in strength, the measures for body composition, maximal oxygen uptake, cardiovascular performance and hemodynamics (related to blood flow) didn't change.

A recent study by J.B. Kramer, et al, from the exercise science department at Appalachian State University in Boone, North Carolina, compared a single set to failure with multiple sets to failure on squat performance. Over the 14-week study, all subjects increased their strength, but the multiple-set group saw about 50% more strength increases than the single-set group.

Naturally, exercise scientists, athletes and coaches want to know what's the most effective way to train. Varying volume (sets and reps), intensity (amount of weight you lift) and frequency of training wins hands down. First and foremost, this means you complete more than one set for each bodypart, which will maximize your body's adaptations in those areas mentioned above. You'll also end up growing stronger and bigger faster. Does this mean single sets to failure have no place in your routine whatsoever? Not at all. Since varying the way you train is key to continued progress, including single sets to failure from time to time would seem appropriate. But do so sparingly, maybe at times when you need to cut short your time in the gym.[5,6]

(**14**)

DIVIDE AND CONQUER

A: Nothing signifies your graduation from beginner to intermediate bodybuilder quite like the day you begin your first split workout. Yup, removing the training wheels from your full-body routine and wobbling on to the infamous chest and arms workout (you know, bench presses and biceps curls for five days straight with weekends off) is a big step — in the wrong direction.

You see, designing the perfect training split is more than just picking and choosing your favorite bodyparts to train. It should not only be balanced and geared toward your specific goals, but it should also change constantly as you monitor your priorities while honestly facing up to your individual strengths and weaknesses. Remember, you have only a finite amount of time and energy to work with every time you step into the gym. If your game plan is poorly designed, those precious resources will go to waste, leaving you with the same muscle-barren body you started with. That said, here's what you need to know to design the best training split for you.

Step 1: Make Time for Recovery

As you progress, a fairly consistent pattern emerges in terms of your general workout split. Shortly after your first workout, you'll add more sets and more exercises, so it becomes imperative that you keep splitting your workout to accommodate the increase in volume. A well-designed split, however, takes more into account than just providing a platform to hammer each muscle group with a high volume of work, then allowing it to recover while you blast other muscle groups on subsequent days. Ask any experienced bodybuilder and he or she will quickly advise you to carefully balance your training with ample rest and recovery time. As you plan your split, know that rest days are just as important as training days. In addition, make sure you're getting enough nutrients throughout the day, and especially after your workout, to refuel energy stores.

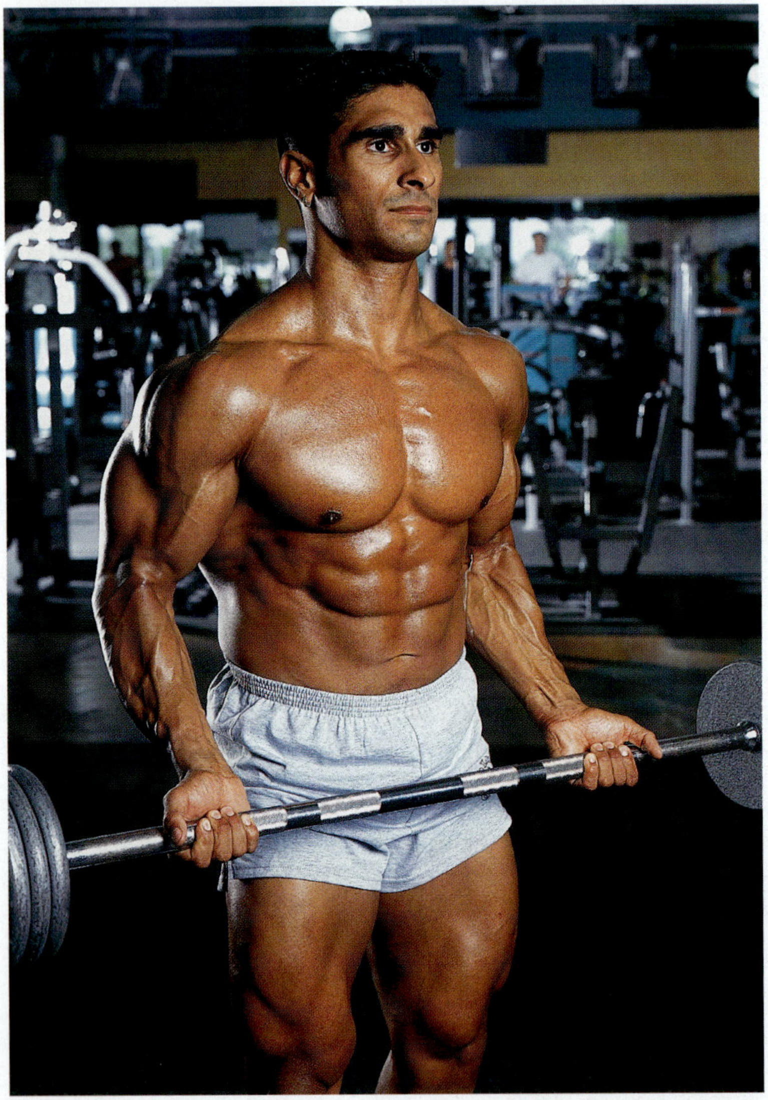

Step 2: Vary Your Intensity

Rest is obviously a key component of the muscle-building process, but there's much more to it than training a different muscle group each day and thinking that the non-working muscles are recovering. If you train at a high level of intensity each time you hit the gym, it doesn't matter if you alternate the muscle groups you train — the cumulative fatigue takes a toll on your energy levels and, subsequently, the degree of muscle growth that can occur.

You'll see the best results in any split routine if you alternate the

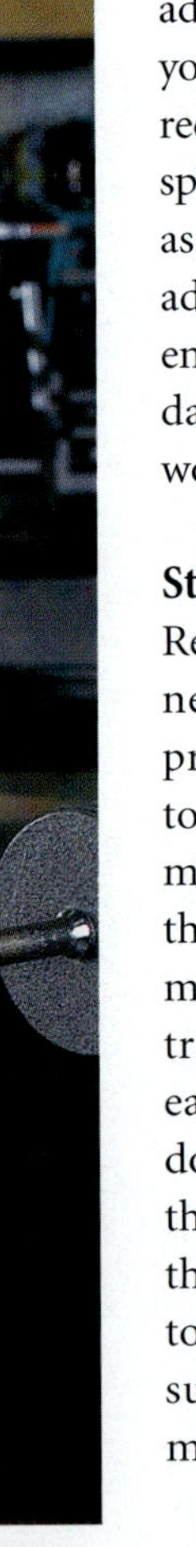

A biceps curl is probably a staple in your routine; do it on an upper body day.

intensity of your workouts as well as the muscle groups you train. That way you can facilitate both muscle repair and recovery of muscle glycogen stores (stored energy) from session to session and week to week. If you reduce the training stimulus to only once per week, you can't possibly develop maximum strength and muscularity. So hitting each muscle group two, maybe even three times, per week with varying intensity is key to maximal gains. Obviously, you'll use more multi-joint movements and fewer exercises and sets in each session. But remember, with 2–3 weekly sessions, you can alternate the exercises you perform to stimulate the

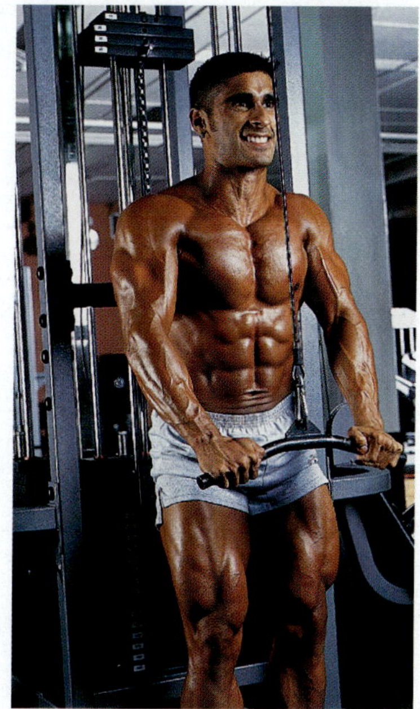

Triceps pressdowns can be done in the push routine of a three-day split.

a two-on, one-off, two-on, two-off program, you're able to hit most muscle groups twice each week, while allowing optimal recovery time for replenishing muscle glycogen and repairing damaged muscle tissue. The most ideal setup would involve the use of a high-intensity workout on day 1, a moderate-intensity workout on day 2, then a full recovery day off. Day 4 would be a moderate-intensity workout, while day 5 is a high-intensity session.

Those who feel they respond better to very high volumes of training might find this structure inadequate for the amount of exercises and sets they want to include for each bodypart. But if

'Designing the perfect training split is more than just picking and choosing your favorite bodyparts to train.'

muscle in a slightly different way each workout, prompting constant gains and assisting in recovery.

Step 3: Choose a Split
Upper body/lower body The first split from a full-body routine is typically a move to separate upper- and lower-body workouts. This effectively cuts your workout time in half, allowing more exercises and more sets for each bodypart to be performed, and you're still able to

stimulate each muscle group twice (in a two-days-on, one-day-off system) or three times per week (alternating workouts for six days with one day off). Either strategy may be effective for general conditioning of the major muscle groups, although training at a high intensity for six days straight may be problematic in terms of energy resource management and recovery.

When this split is performed as

you've been hitting each bodypart once per week with a high volume of training for any length of time, you're probably a prime candidate for this type of split.

Three-day split (push/pull/legs) If you're like most trainees, you probably tried an upper-/ lower-body split early on, but as you continued to add more exercises to your upper-body day, this workout soon required double the time of the legs day and

'Be sure to train larger bodyparts like back and legs before smaller bodyparts like arms on a given day.'

another split had to be made.

The three-day split has many forms. Like other multiday splits, you could potentially put any combination of muscle groups together to compose the three separate workouts. The most common three-day routines, however, are based on a modified push/pull/legs system. This often employs a bevy of multijoint movements and one full day of rest between each workout, for example: legs (squats, front squats, leg presses, lunges, step-ups) on Monday, pushing movements (presses, dips, arm extensions) on Wednesday and pulling movements (deadlifts, rows, pull-ups, pull-downs, arm curls) on Friday.

Alternatively, this can be done as a three-day rotation followed by a rest day. This system allows you to hit each bodypart almost twice per week, but if you're training at a high intensity 5–6 days weekly without cycling the intensity of your workouts, overtraining will inevitably lead to a plateau. Alternating workouts with days off will ensure you're adequately rested before each high-intensity session. (But as indicated earlier,

stimulating each bodypart only once each week may not provide optimal results.)

When it comes to possible splits on a 4–5-day program, variety isn't a problem. You can go as far as doing one bodypart per day (chest, back, shoulders, legs and arms, for example) or you can combine bodyparts, anything from back and triceps to shoulders and abs. Just be sure to train larger bodyparts like back and legs before smaller bodyparts like arms on a given day, especially in the case of triceps before shoulders or chest, or biceps before back.

Choose a split based on your own schedule and level of training expertise. If you're still relatively new to training, it's probably best to start with the upper-/lower-body split and progress down the list every few months or so. Keep in mind, however, that just because you may be an advanced bodybuilder doesn't mean you should never see a two- or three-day split in your workout log again. By varying the intensity and volume of your training, you can make

every one of these splits work for you, no matter what your level of experience. Relatively frequent alterations to your training split will keep your muscles growing and your strength improving.

THE FORMULA FOR SUCCESS

I typically see intensity and volume listed in descriptions of workouts. Can you define these and explain how they interact to elicit desired training outcomes?

A: Defining intensity and volume isn't a simple task, as different sources offer varied explanations. The parameters that compose these terms are more concrete, however, so even though the terminology may be somewhat ambiguous, the big picture is clearer. Understanding the relationship between intensity and volume will help you realize why they're crucial elements to your training.

Intense Relations

Intensity is directly related to 1RM — the greatest resistance you can lift once, and only once, for a given movement. The intensity increases as the weight of an exercise approaches your 1RM. Furthermore, intensity is dependent upon time — the time between reps, sets and exercises. As rest time decreases, intensity increases.

Rest between sets is critical, but some leeway exists within the recommended range of 30 seconds to three minutes (60–90 seconds is the norm). Generally, the heavier you train, the longer you need to rest if your goal is maximum recovery between each set. Rest between reps is more difficult to change, but you can alter your lifting speed somewhat without losing control. Slight changes in rest time, whether it's between sets or reps, can have a dramatic effect on the intensity of a workout and the muscle pump you experience.

Pumping up the Volume

Training volume can be thought of as the total work performed or the total weight lifted. A simple way to measure volume is to multiply the exercise resistance by the number of repetitions and the number

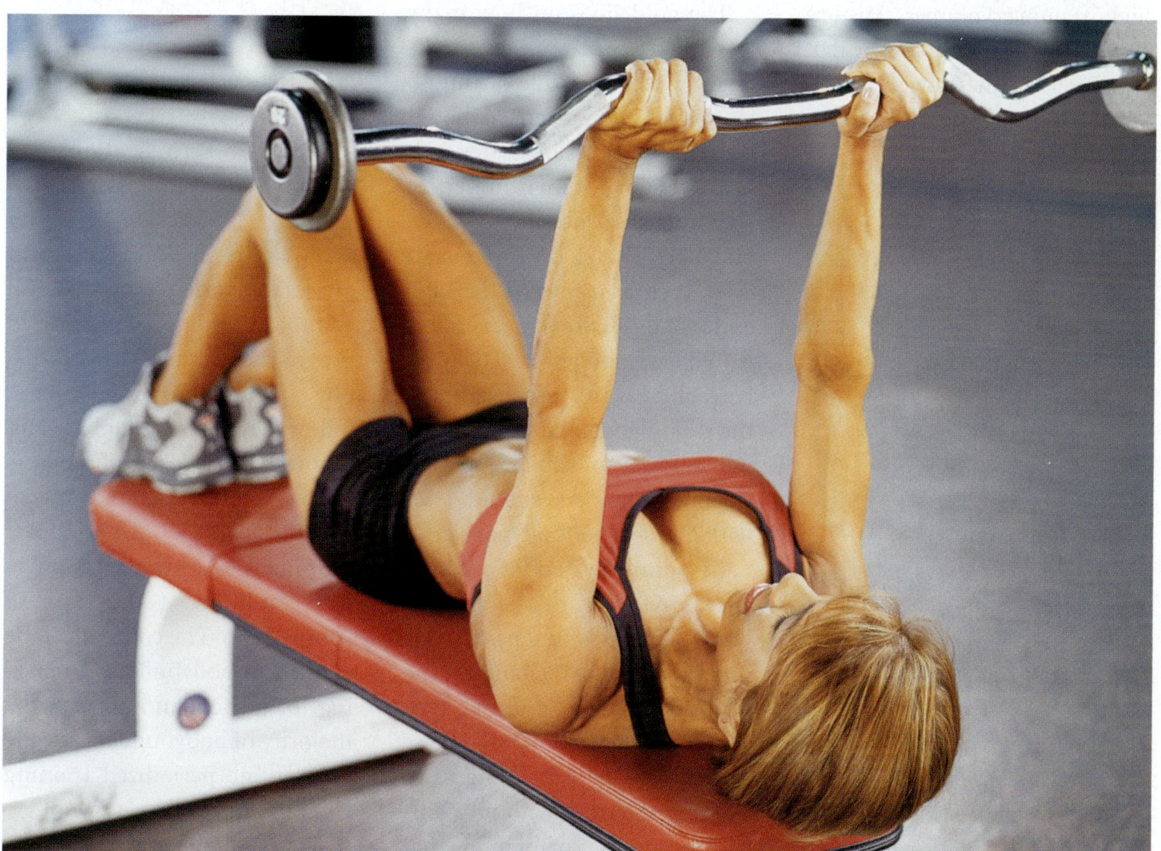

To raise the intensity of a movement, increase resistance or decrease rest time. To increase volume, add more reps and/or sets.

of sets (weight x reps x sets). At first glance, it appears that an unlimited number of values can be computed for training volume. Yet decades of research have provided optimal training parameters for developing size. The guessing game is reduced to a reliable method of plugging the right numbers into the equation.

Why Failure is Good

Bodybuilding mandates the use of high training volumes. History and experience have shown that repetitions in the range of 6–10 are best suited for increasing mus-

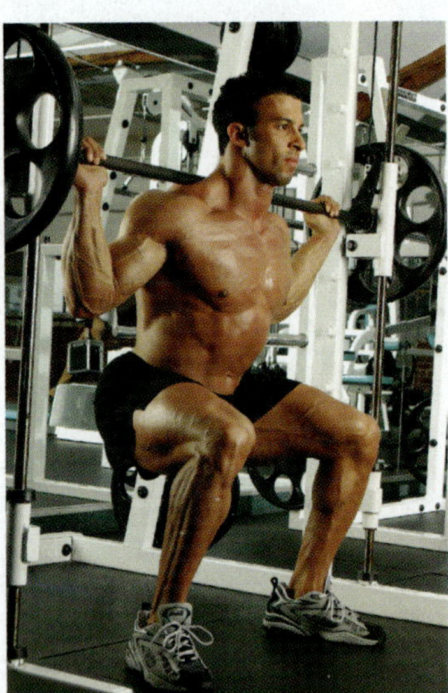

Choose a resistance that allows you to perform six to 10 repetitions.

cle size and strength. Likewise, training to failure is an excellent way to stimulate muscle hypertrophy by fatiguing a maximum number of muscle fibers. Of course, the most successful bodybuilders learn what works best for them by manipulating the intensity and volume of their workouts. Hence, choosing a training resistance that allows at least six but no more than 10 reps will not only provide the best training stimulus but also completes the first two blanks of the volume equation. The only remaining value is the number of sets.

The guidelines on how many sets to perform aren't as well-established, but a rule of thumb is 3–5 sets for advanced bodybuilders. Of course, this depends somewhat on the number of exercises you do for a given bodypart. If you do three exercises, then lean toward the high end (five sets); five exercises would warrant fewer sets (perhaps three). In both examples, the training volume is comparable — 15 sets of similar reps and weight. Beginners should start with 6–9 sets per bodypart.

In summary, adding resistance or reducing rest periods (or both) increases intensity. Volume is altered by changing the resistance, reps and/or sets. Minor modifications to these parameters cause changes in training intensity without compromising the principles that build muscle mass.

16

THE STAGES OF SUCCESS

I've trained fairly heavy for years, but I recently read that cycling my program can actually deliver better results. What is periodization and how can it benefit me as a bodybuilder?

A: Periodization is a term used to describe training that's broken into phases of varied intensity and volume. A traditional periodized program consists of a hypertrophy (muscle-building) phase, followed by a strength phase and a power phase; each phase lasts from several weeks to a couple of months. The goal of periodized training is to achieve peak physical condition at the time of competition. The concept can be applied to bodybuilders preparing for a show and, in fact, the majority of bodybuilders already incorporate periodized training whether they realize it or not.

Most athletes require power to elicit maximal performance.

'Training to failure is an excellent way to stimulate muscle hypertrophy by fatiguing a maximum number of muscle fibers.'

Although power is important for bodybuilders, mass is the ultimate goal. Therefore, the phase sequence of periodized training is different — practically reversed — from that of the power athlete. Minimal power training will preface a moderate strength phase. The major focus becomes building size in the third segment. A fourth stage of diet, cardio and reduced intensity helps shed bodyfat and enhance definition just before a competition.

Power Phase

This phase is characterized by high intensity (2–4 reps max (RM); a weight that's heavy enough to allow only 2–4 repetitions) and low volume (total number of reps performed per workout session). The power phase is useful for introducing occasional variety and shocking the muscles into growth but isn't a critical component of periodized training for bodybuilders. If utilized, it should be undertaken only after a solid foundation of muscle conditioning has been established.

Strength Phase

The intensity decreases moving into the strength phase (4–6 RM), but more repetitions lead to an increase in volume, with number of sets and exercises remaining

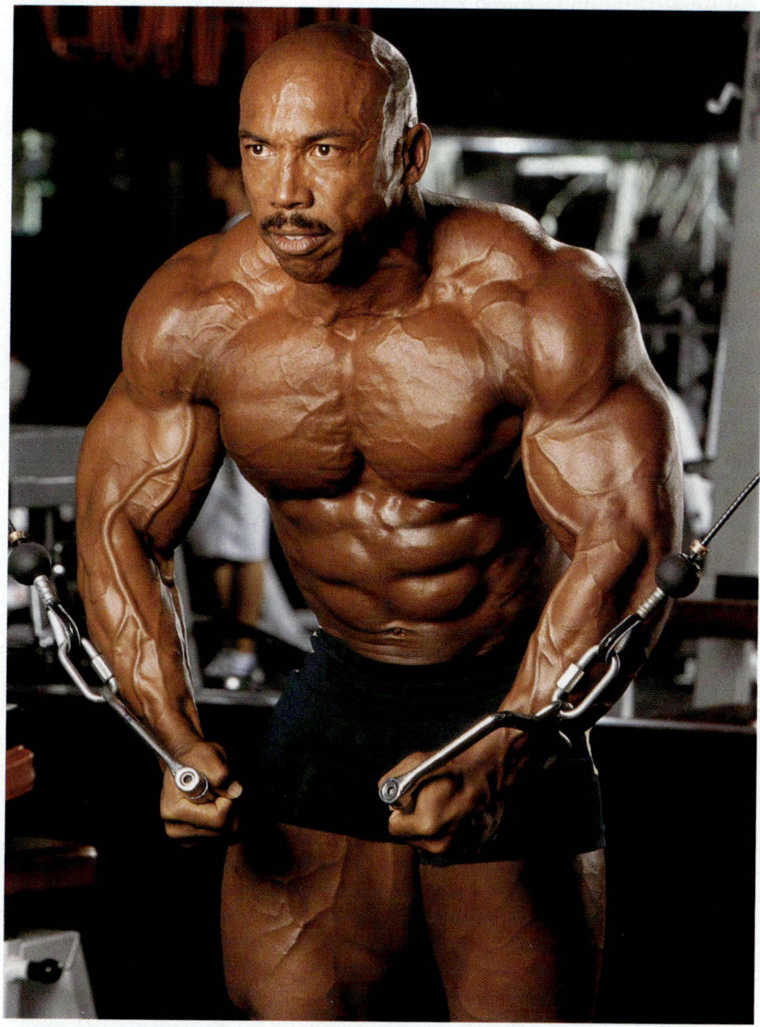

During the hypertrophy phase, training volume increases as intensity decreases.

constant. Spend a moderate amount of time in this phase — at least a few weeks, but no more than two months.

Mass Phase

The hypertrophy, or mass phase, should be the backbone of your periodized training program and comprise at least half of the total training time. (If you start the periodized training regimen six months before a contest, the hypertrophy phase should last 3–4 months.) Training volume continues to increase as intensity decreases (6–10 RM). Use the strength you've gained to build some serious mass.

Precontest Phase

Some bodybuilders can transition from the hypertrophy phase to competition in a week or less. It depends upon several variables including genetics, nutrition, water retention, etc. If you find it difficult to get cut up, you'll need to spend more time in this fourth and final stage. Intensity can be further decreased (10–15 RM), but isn't a necessity. The crucial component is diet. Aerobic activity can also be helpful to promote fat loss.

Trial and error will help you decide how much time to spend in each phase of periodized training. Nothing is written in stone and nothing is for certain, with one possible exception: Nothing encourages continued muscle growth better than variety, and altering training volume and intensity is one of the best ways to enhance the muscle-building stimulus.

17

YOUR MAX LIFT

What does "1RM" mean, and how is it important in bodybuilding?

A: The abbreviation 1RM represents one-repetition maximum, the heaviest resistance you can lift for one complete repetition of an exercise using good form.[7] Although 1RM movements are common among powerlifters and other athletes training for power, such lifts aren't customary for bodybuilders who want to gain mass. But the 1RM is still an important bodybuilding tool for measuring strength and designing training programs.

The concept of repetition maximum (RM) isn't used exclusively for single-repetition sets. In fact, the RM system is most frequently used for sets of multiple repetitions. The expanded, general definition for RM is "the maximum weight you can lift for a given number of reps." If you're squatting, for example, using every last ounce of energy to squeeze out seven reps, you've just done a 7RM set of squats. Therefore, every time you push a set to failure, you're performing an RM.

The consensus among bodybuilders is that exercising to failure is key to packing on muscle. Going to failure not only fatigues more muscle fibers but also requires maximal motor neuron recruitment. In short, greater muscle involvement leads to fuller

'Going to failure not only fatigues more muscle fibers but also requires maximal motor neuron recruitment.'

development. Exercising to failure is most beneficial, however, when the number of repetitions falls within a desired

Estimating One-Repetition Maximum

Repetitions:	1	2	3	4	5	6	7	8	9	10
Weight lifted (lbs.):	50	47	45	44	43	42	40	39	38	37
	60	56	55	53	52	50	48	47	45	44
	70	65	64	62	60	58	56	55	53	50
	80	75	73	70	69	67	65	63	60	58
	90	84	82	80	77	75	73	70	68	65
	100	93	91	88	86	83	81	78	76	73
	110	105	100	97	95	92	90	86	83	80
	120	112	110	105	103	100	97	95	90	85
	130	125	120	115	110	108	105	100	98	95
	140	130	128	125	120	117	113	110	105	100
	150	140	136	133	130	125	120	118	115	110
	160	150	145	140	137	133	130	125	120	117
	170	160	155	150	145	140	137	133	130	125
	180	170	165	160	155	150	145	140	135	130
	190	180	175	170	165	160	155	150	145	140
	200	190	185	180	175	170	165	160	155	150
	210	195	190	185	180	175	170	165	160	155
	220	205	200	195	190	185	180	175	170	165
	230	215	210	205	195	190	185	180	175	170
	240	225	220	210	205	200	195	190	185	175
	250	235	225	220	215	210	200	195	190	185
	260	245	235	230	225	220	210	205	200	190
	270	250	245	240	235	225	220	210	205	200
	280	260	255	245	240	235	225	220	215	205
	290	270	265	255	250	245	235	230	220	215
	300	280	275	265	260	250	245	235	230	220
	310	290	280	275	265	260	250	245	235	230
	320	300	290	285	275	270	260	250	245	235
	330	310	300	290	285	275	265	260	250	245
	340	315	310	300	295	285	275	265	260	250
	350	330	320	310	300	295	285	275	265	260
	360	335	330	320	310	300	290	280	275	265
	370	345	335	325	320	310	300	290	280	270
	380	355	345	335	325	320	310	300	290	280
	390	365	355	345	335	325	315	305	295	285
	400	375	365	355	345	335	325	315	305	295

Adapted and modified from *Essentials of Strength Training and Conditioning* by the National Strength and Conditioning Association, Thomas R. Baechle, ed. Copyright 1994 by the National Strength and Conditioning Association. Excerpted by permission of Human Kinetics, Champaign, IL. Second edition, June 2000, available in bookstores or by calling 800-747-4457. $59 plus s/h.

Most of you probably don't know exactly what you can lift for one rep on the exercises you typically do. Use this chart only as an approximation of what you could do, and don't be thrown off by the poundages you can't really put on the bar — just round up or down. As an example, if you can bench press 205 pounds for five reps, find the five-rep column and go down to 205. Next, go all the way to the left until you're in the one-rep column; you'll see that 240 is your approximate 1RM.

range. The magic number for bodybuilders is in the range of about 6–10 reps.

To lift and reach muscle failure in a 6–10-rep range, you must first select the proper resistance. If you're a seasoned veteran, experience makes this a trivial task. For the novice bodybuilder or those who prefer training with a scientific slant, charts have been developed to determine the correct weight for achieving the desired number of reps (based on your 1RM).[8] Conversely, if you know how many max reps you can do with a given resistance, the charts will furnish your 1RM.

Besides serving as a baseline to gauge workout weights, the 1RM is a good measure of muscular strength and is used regularly in clinical settings. For bodybuilders, it's a good

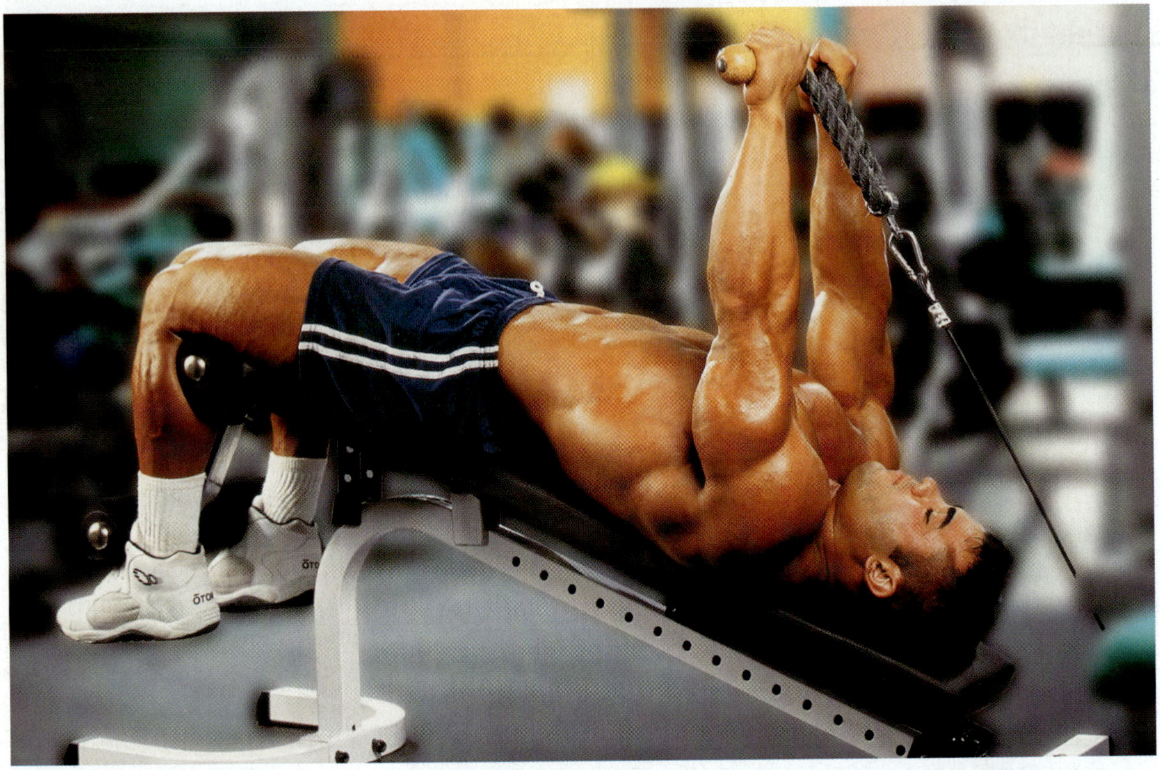

By slightly adjusting the angle at which you perform an exercise, you will force muscles to contract in different ways.

idea to do a 1RM strength test every 1–3 months for core exercises. This provides feedback regarding strength gains and updates your 1RM reference point for calculating rep weights.

Precede a 1RM strength test with an adequate warm-up and include no more than five attempts, separated by at least three-minute rest intervals. More attempts or less rest may lead to inaccurate results because of fatigue. As you become more experienced, accurately finding your 1RM will become a simple task.

Use the RM system to take some of the guesswork out of your workouts and to provide yourself with valuable training data. The frequent use of 1RM sets won't elicit desirable results for the average bodybuilder, but occasional use will not only stimulate your muscles in a new way but also provide insight into the effectiveness of your training.

18

THE BEST OF BOTH WORLDS

Is it best to change my workout every time I go to the gym, or should I stick with the routine I've been using that seems to deliver results?

'On the other side of the spectrum, lighten the load occasionally and bump up the reps to 12–20.'

A: One of the finer arts of bodybuilding is sifting through the numerous exercises and techniques to find what works best for you. On one hand, you're grateful to have finally put together a winning routine, and therefore reluctant to mess it up. On the other hand, you know that variety is what makes training fun and keeps your muscles growing. So why not do both?

Of course, you can't strictly do both, but with a little give and take, maybe you can have the best of both worlds. Start by keeping your time-tested routine; it will form the backbone of your new program. Next, make a subtle change, whether it's the resistance, number of reps or the exercise order. Now you have your new routine, only it's your old routine with a twist.

Here are some changes you can make to keep your workouts fresh while maintaining or even increasing their effectiveness.

Try going ultra-heavy once in a while to shock your muscles. Keep the reps in the 3–6 range and don't forget to rest a little longer between sets. On the other side of the spectrum, lighten the load occasionally and bump up the reps to 12–20. The change will be refreshing and your tired body will welcome the reduced load. Whether you go heavy or light, your training volume should stay about the same (volume = reps x weight).

Movement Angle: Small variations in the angle at which a muscle is stressed can make a tremendous difference in the way it responds. You may think you're simply moving the bench a few degrees when you do your bench press at a slight incline, but your pecs believe that you've discovered a new exercise. Your chest will be stimulated in a new way, forcing it to contract differently than what it's accustomed to. Whether you change your foot placement, grip width or bench angle, or substitute a cable exercise for the free-weight version, modest changes give way to more significant changes in growth.

Change the order. In theory, changing the order of your exercises doesn't really alter your routine. After all, you're using the same movements and doing the same amount of work. Yet it does change the way in which your muscles fatigue, and thus stresses them in a different way. If you always do bench presses first, then you're somewhat weaker on your successive exercises. Do inclines first next time. This is probably the quickest and easiest way to change your routine without making significant modifications.

You can probably come up with some other ways to modify your training without changing the underlying framework. Be creative in developing new workouts and always remember to make training fun.

STAND UP, SIT DOWN

If an exercise can be performed in a seated or a standing position, which is better for developing strength and mass?

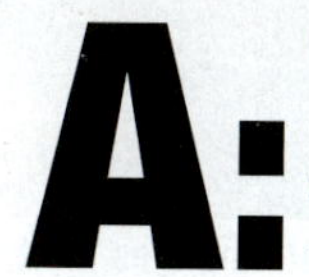

A: Each position — seated and standing — offers certain benefits. The

'The stabilizing muscles called upon during standing exercises contribute to the development of the hip, abdominal and lower back muscles.'

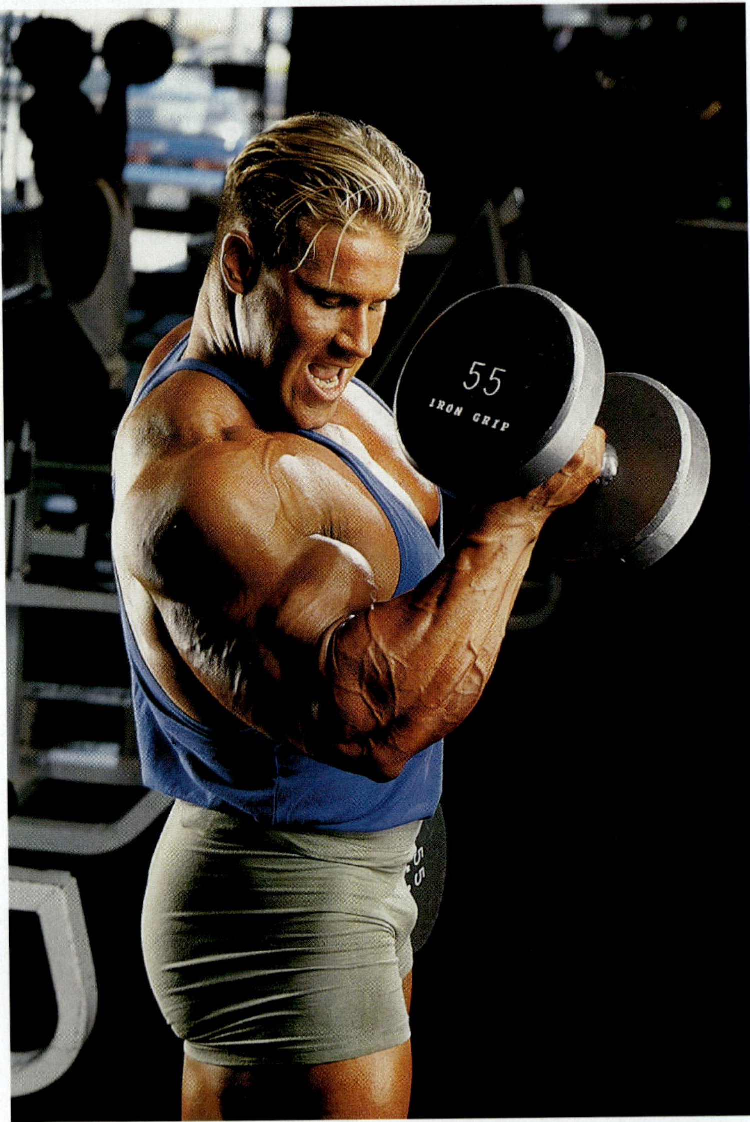

A standing dumbbell curl engages more working muscles than a seated one.

exercise mechanics are slightly different for each, changing the movement enough to stimulate the target muscle in a different way. Although seemingly insignificant, minor modifications can have a significant impact on overall muscle development. The position that works best for you may depend upon your training goals, muscle response or simply personal preference.

Of the exercises that can be performed seated or standing, most are upper-body movements. Shoulder moves include the overhead press, front raise, lateral raise and even the bent-over lateral raise. Many of the assorted biceps dumbbell exercises, like alternating dumbbell curls and hammer curls, can be performed seated or standing. Overhead triceps extensions and kickbacks are triceps movements that can be done from either position.

Taking a Seat

The primary advantage of performing exercises from a seated position is that the lower body is essentially eliminated from the movement, shifting emphasis toward the working muscle. This enables better isolation and the ability to concentrate on a smaller area of contracting muscle. Bodybuilders wishing to target a specific muscle group may find this useful.

Keeping the lower body stable is generally safer, because of the improved support of the lower back and torso — especially notable for athletes who suffer from back problems. It's also more difficult to cheat on certain movements by using body momentum to get a weight up.

Taking a Stand

Exercising from a standing position offers two distinct advantages: 1) you can often handle more weight and 2) it incorporates a greater number of working muscles (legs, hips and torso) to keep the body stabilized and upright. Moving more weight means two things: more mass and greater strength. Enough said.

Whether you'll benefit from the involvement of stabilizers and assisting muscles (muscles other than the intended muscle group) is a more controversial subject. At first glance, using muscles beyond those required for exercise execution seems counterproductive. For bodybuilders purely after larg-

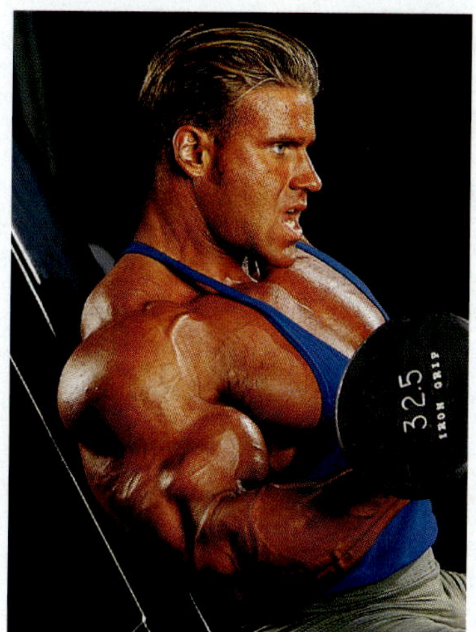

Sitting results in concentration on a smaller area of contracted muscle.

er muscles for aesthetic purposes, such an argument might hold some weight, but certainly not in the case of athletes in other sports. The strength required in many athletic endeavors stems from the torso. The stabilizing muscles called upon during standing exercises contribute to the development of the hip, abdominal and lower back muscles, and that strength transfers directly to success in many different activities.

The Winner Is . . .

When it comes right down to it, neither position is inherently better than the other. You should regularly perform exercises in both positions to introduce vari-

ety into your training and stress your muscles from as many angles as possible. By using both positions, you'll reap the benefits of each. In this instance, you can have your cake and eat it, too!

20

BUILDING HUGE WHEELS

For whatever reason, my legs lag behind my upper body. I like to pre-exhaust my legs before I squat by doing 3–4 sets of seven reps of leg curls followed by the same number of leg extensions. Then I squat 225 pounds for three sets of about seven reps. I do this once a week. What am I doing wrong? I just want a huge set of wheels.

A:
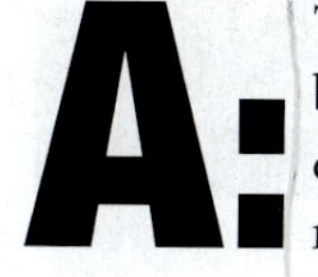
The key to remember is that you can't develop quality muscle unless you

'You can't develop quality muscle unless you lift heavy weight. Focus primarily on getting stronger.'

lift heavy weight. This means your primary focus should be on getting stronger. As you grow stronger, a welcome byproduct is larger muscles. Now, does this mean that you need to do singles, doubles and triples like many powerlifters and weightlifters do? No, not exactly. Must you load up your squat to 315 and take it for all it's worth right now? Nope. What you need to do is progressively increase the weight you use and decrease your rep range to about five.

Here's how you might go about it, remembering that you should take it slow and not hope to have 30-inch thighs by next month. The primary thing you should do is squat first in your workout. This exercise should become the backbone of your quad training. Next, up the volume for each of your exercises to five sets and replace the leg extensions with leg presses, lunges or step-ups. Also add another movement to your hamstrings workout such as standing leg curls, Romanian deadlifts or glute-ham raises.

As far as the whole workout goes, go up in intensity (amount of weight you lift) equally on all your exercises every other week. The following week, go back down to the weights you typically use (for example, 225 pounds in the squat). Keep using this increase-decrease protocol until you reach a weight that you can't squat for three reps on your heavy day. At that point, take a week off and start over,

but now your 225-pound weeks become 230 pounds and you increase the weight you lift during your heavy weeks by 5 pounds, too. Here's how it might look for the squat:

Week	Weight	Reps (estimate)
1	225	7
2	235	6
3	225	7
4	245	6
5	225	7
6	255	5
7	225	7
8	265	4
9	225	7
10	275	3

21

TRAINING SPECIFICITY

I'm really into body-building and I think lifting has helped me in other sports, too. But here's my question: If I want to get more of a performance boost, do I need to change the way I bodybuild?

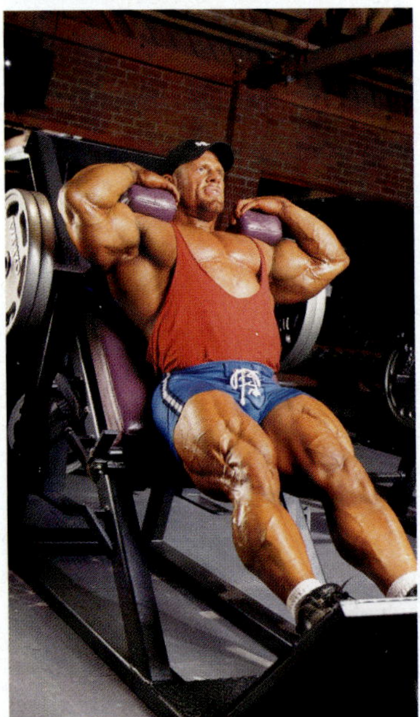

Do hack squats early in your workout.

A: The way you body-build will impact your sport performance. The key variable you need to consider is training specificity — gearing your bodybuilding to match the specifics of your sport. How important is training specificity? Check out the research.

When S. McCaw and J. Friday from the Biomechanics Laboratory at Illinois State University in Normal compared the free-weight and machine bench press, they found that the muscular activity generated in the free-weight bench press was significantly greater than in the machine bench press. The implication is that improving your machine bench press won't improve your strength in a free-weight bench press, nor can you expect as much growth development. Similarly, T.G. Chandler, et al, from Northeast Missouri State University in Kirksville examined the lat pull-down and pull-up, concluding that each exercise was sufficiently different to preclude strength comparisons.

To round things off, G. Wilson and colleagues from the Centre for Exercise Science & Sport Management at Southern Cross University in

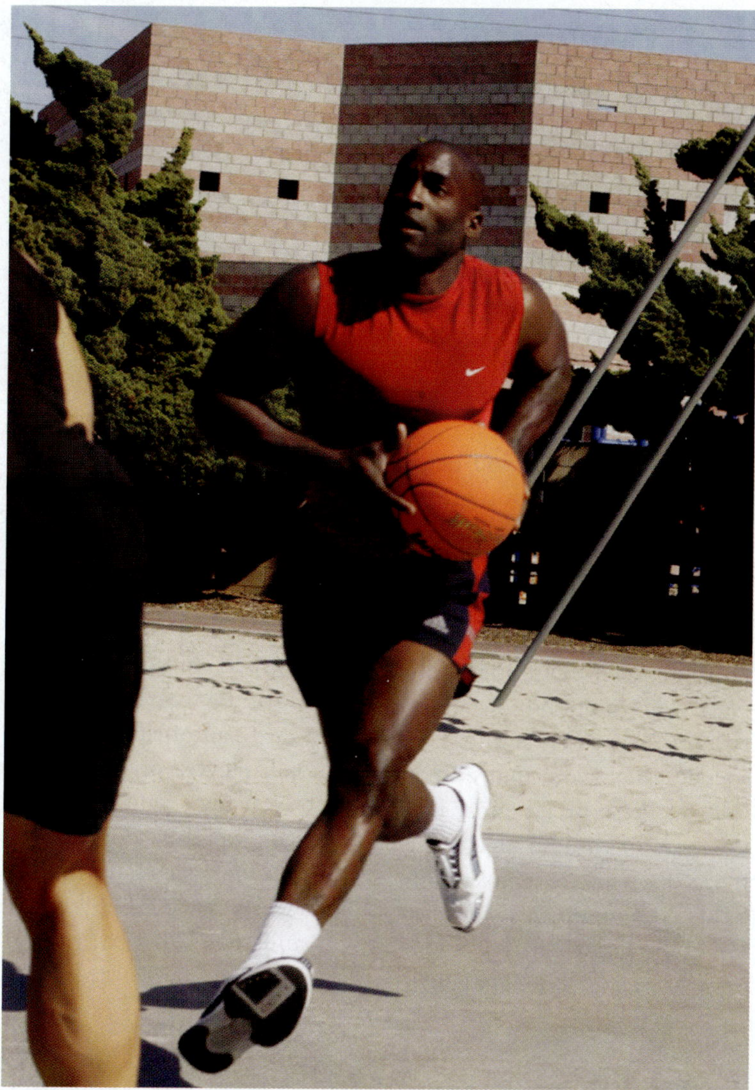

A basketball player might work high-speed bodybuilding into his training.

Lismore, Australia, found that when it comes to plyometrics and strength training, the plyos significantly enhance eccentric lower-body force production; weightlifting will enhance the concentric portion. They conclude that these results are due to the different and specific stresses placed on the body by each form of exercise.

So what does this mean for

'Determine what kind of demands your sport places on your body, whether endurance, power, or speed.'

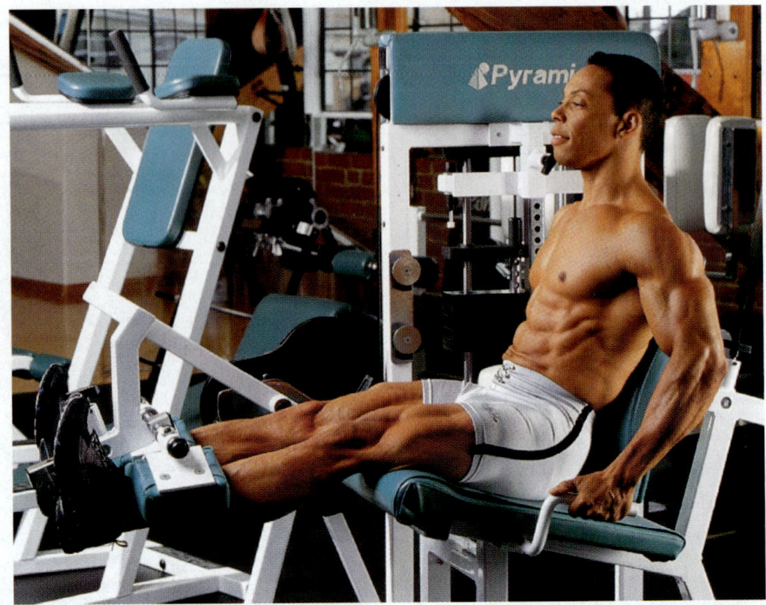

No matter what sport you play, bodybuilding is essential to developing strength.

your training? First, you need to bodybuild to develop greater strength in any sport. Second, you need to train for the specific demands of your sport. First determine what kind of demands your sport places on your body, whether endurance, power, strength or speed. Once you figure that out, decide how it's most important for you to maximize that skill. If you're a boxer with fights coming up this summer, for example, you may want to emphasize lighter-weight bench presses and military presses, but move the weight explosively and with authority. If you're a football player, on the other hand, you may want to lift the heaviest weights possible to bulk up and get ready for the next season. Accordingly, your sets and reps will vary, too. In the first example, do more sets per bodypart and 10–15 reps. In the second example, do 5–8 sets per bodypart and 3–5 reps.

As specific as our bodies are, bodybuilding will be a key in your sport-specific development. If you use an intelligent approach that can pinpoint your specific demands, you're on the right track. ■

References

1. American College of Sports Medicine. The recommended quantity and quality of exercise for developing and maintaining cardiorespiratory and muscular fitness, and flexibility in healthy adults. Medicine & Science in Sports & Exercise 30(5):975–991, 1998.

2. Braith, R.W., et al. Comparison of two vs. three days per week of variable resistance training during 10- and 18-week programs. International Journal of Sports Medicine 10:450–454, 1989.

3. Dudley, G.A., et al. Importance of eccentric actions in performance adaptations to resistance training. Aviation Space and Environmental Medicine 62:543–550, 1991.

4. Feigenbaum, M.S., Pollock, M.L. Strength training: rationale for current guidelines for adult fitness programs. Physician and Sportsmedicine 25:44–64, 1997. 5) Fleck, S., Kraemer, W. Designing resistance training programs. Champaign, IL: Human Kinetics, 1997. 6) Komi, P.V. Strength and power in sport. Cambridge, MA: Blackwell Science, 1992.

5. Hurley, B.F. Effects of high-intensity strength training on cardiovascular function. Medicine & Science in Sports & Exercise 16(5):483–488, 1984.

6. Kramer, J.B., et al. Effects of single vs. multiple sets of weight training: impact of volume, intensity and variation. Journal of Strength & Conditioning Research 11(3):143–147, 1997.

7. Fleck, S.J., Kraemer, W.J. Designing resistance training programs. (2nd ed.) Champaign, IL: Human Kinetics, 1997.

8. Wathen, D. Load assignment. In: Essentials of strength training and conditioning. Champaign, IL: Human Kinetics, 1994.

9. Chandler, T.G., et al. Relationship of pull-up and lat-pull performances to 1RM lat-pull strength. Journal of Strength and Conditioning Research 9(3):205, 1995.

10. McCaw, S., Friday, J. A comparison of muscle activity between a free weight and machine bench press. Journal of Strength and Conditioning Research 8(4):259–264, 1994.

11. Wilson, G., et al. Weight and plyometric training: Effects on eccentric and concentric force production. Canadian Journal of Applied Physiology 21(4):301–315, 1996.

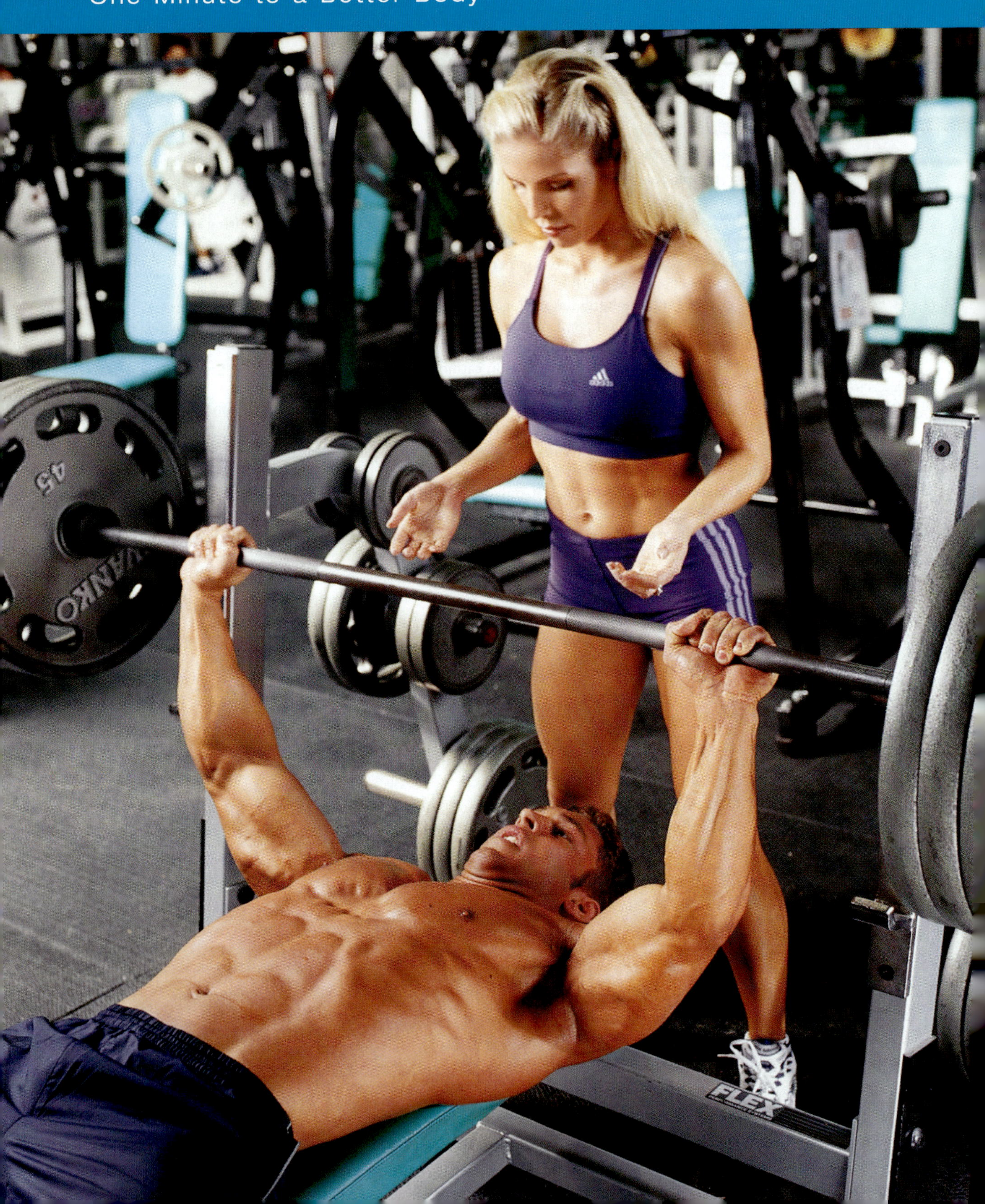

PERFECT FORM

Lifting techniques for safe and effective gains

Next time you're working out, use one of your rest periods to take a long, lingering look around the weight room. Chances are you'll see a wide variety of lifting "techniques" on display — in all their hilarity. There's the spaghetti-armed teen flapping his arms in the mirror, using all available momentum to finish a punishing set of lat raises. And the grunting woman on the foam mat, locking her hands behind her head and forcefully pulling up to complete her crunches. And then there's that big fellow, splayed on a bench with a barbell squashing his stomach, heaving up and down to exercise his abs. No, really.

With this kind of craziness going on, you're likely to conclude, correctly, that there's an epidemic of bad technique running through the gyms and

'There are right and wrong ways to move the weight, avoid injury and stimulate muscle fibers.'

health clubs of America. But let's make one thing clear: All of us, no matter how many years we've toiled in the weight room, can stand to revisit our understanding of lifting techniques.

And that's what this section is for — to clear up the doubts and questions, both fundamental and obscure, that can occasionally creep into your head and throw off your training progress. With every resistance exercise, there are right and wrong ways to move the weight, avoid injury and stimulate muscle fibers toward maximal growth. However, not all of these are common knowledge. For instance, did you know that holding your breath through the sticking point of a movement could allow you to be 20% stronger? Or that you should use a weight belt sparingly, saving it for your heaviest lifts? Or that it's usually dangerous techniques — not dangerous movements — that lead to injury?

These realities, and many more, are revealed and fully explained over the next several pages. But before you dive into that bubbling pool of eye-opening information, here are a few key concepts to

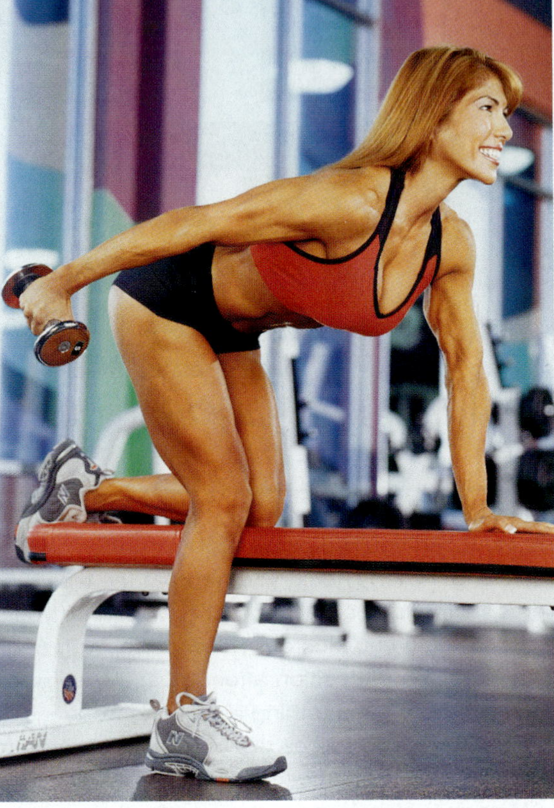

keep in mind during every single repetition that you perform, no matter what the exercise:

Breathe right. Though resistance training is anaerobic in nature, meaning the energy your body uses to lift weights comes from a stored source that doesn't require oxygen to release energy, you can't just hold your breathe throughout movements. The general rule of thumb is to exhale on the positive portion of the rep (lifting the weight) and inhale on the negative portion (lowering the weight). You should be able to take deeper-than-normal breaths; if you can squeeze in only quick gasps during your reps, you're probably moving too quickly. For more details, see "Exhale After Exertion," page 62.

Pace yourself. Each rep should be done under control through a deliberate cadence. Swing a weight too fast and momentum takes over to bear the load instead of the intended muscles, sometimes putting your joints at risk. See "Speed & Gains," page 70, for more.

Visualize the exercise. Many successful body-builders attest that training is as much mental as it is physical. Focusing on the target muscle relaxing and contracting to move the resistance will help you not only move more weight but also do more reps. As you curl a dumbbell, for example, see your biceps contracting to pull the weight toward your shoulder. Taking the time to perform this mental exercise will help you develop a mind-muscle link, giving you a control over your body you never thought possible.

Recognize pain. In bodybuilding, there are two distinct types of pain: the pain caused by doing an exercise incorrectly or with too much weight (bad pain), and the pain associated with a burning sensation in the muscle, as the fibers fatigue and lactic acid builds up (good pain). If an exercise is causing pain in your joints, a tearing sensation, or just feels awkward even after numerous sets and reps done with correct form, don't continue with it. Everybody is built somewhat differently, so what feels right to your training partner may not feel right to you. Learn to differentiate good pain from bad, and modify your program based on what works for you.

Now, on to the Q & As. Study them with care, and soon you'll be the smartest, safest, best lifter in your gym — a shining example of perfect form and a powerful vaccine in the never-ending battle against the bad-technique epidemic. More power — and muscle — to you.

Perfect Form: Questions and Answers

SPINAL ALIGNMENT

I've had some lower back problems in the past and want to avoid aggravating this area while still training hard. What do you recommend?

A: Lower back injury is a common problem affecting people from all walks of life, including bodybuilders. Injury stems from any number of circumstances, but most problems are avoidable. The secret is in the curvature of the spine. Without proper curvature, exercise efficiency plummets while the risk of injury increases.

Your spine is an intricate structure. It's sturdy enough to house and protect the spinal cord, yet it's flexible enough to permit movement in all directions. The elastic intervertebral discs, which serve as shock absorbers between the vertebrae, allow spinal mobility while maintaining a high degree of stability. But these discs are susceptible to injury when they're subjected to high compressive forces or put into compromising positions.

When in a "neutral" position, your spine has a natural S-shaped curve, and the discs can withstand tremendous amounts of force. Deviation from neutral alignment — whether from spinal flexion, extension, rotation or a combination thereof — causes disc compression in a non-uniform manner, leading to excessive compression on one side of the disc and/or extreme bulging on the opposite side.

Even under unloaded conditions (no additional weight added), the weight of the head and upper body is significant enough to cause disc damage. Exercise exacerbates the problem, with added resistance significantly increasing the compressive and shearing forces placed upon the spine.

Reduce the Risk

To reduce your risk of back injury, you should: 1) keep your spine in neutral alignment (or as close to it as possible), especially when exercising, but also as you go about your regular daily activities and 2) keep your torso muscles (abdominals and lower back) well-conditioned to support your spine and keep it aligned. Additionally, use good body mechanics when lifting or bending, and use a weight belt sparingly, reserving it only for your heaviest lifts.

Keeping your back in proper position becomes increasingly difficult as you progress from seated with backrest support, to seated unsupported, and on to standing, lying down or an exercise position somewhere in between. If you learn to adopt neutral spine alignment while standing, through practice you can easily transfer it to other positions.

Align Yourself for Success

The key to neutral alignment starts with the head. If you look down, your neck bends, often followed by rounding of the shoulders, ultimately leading to rounding of the back. As you can see, a simple mistake at one end

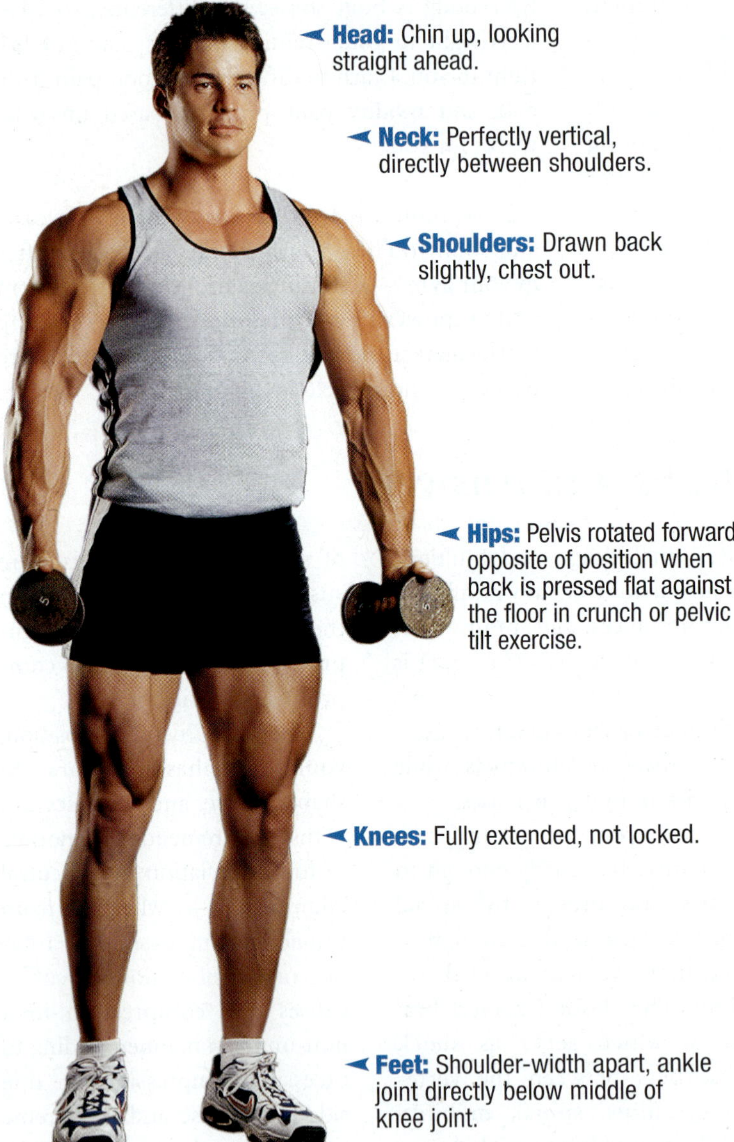

of the spine can translate into dramatic misalignment farther down the line. As a general rule, neutral alignment is achieved when the head, neck, shoulder joint, hip joint, knee joint and ankle joint form a straight, vertical line when viewed from the side. The checklist at left will help you get everything in place to attain neutral alignment when standing.

23

GOING 'ROUND THE BEND

I often read that I should bend at the hips instead of the waist when performing certain exercises. What's the difference?

A: Although seemingly similar, bending at the waist and bending at the hips are two entirely different movements. Each is appropriate for specific exercises. Knowing when and where to bend is necessary for proper exercise performance and injury prevention.

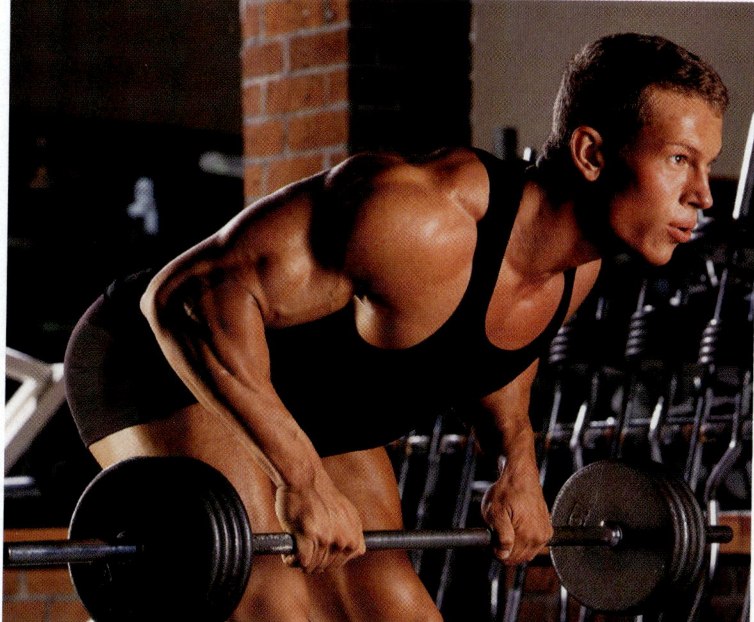
When doing the bent-over barbell row, you should always bend at the hips.

Shooting From the Hip

As a general rule, bending should always come from the hips, not the waist. Bending at the hips (hip flexion) requires that your upper body remain fixed, with all movement restricted to the hip joint formed by the femur and pelvis. The spine should not bend: You must keep it in its normal, neutral alignment, as when sitting or standing with your back straight. Bending at the hips changes your center of gravity, altering your balance. You'll need to stick your glutes out and bend your knees, depending upon the exercise, to keep from falling over.

The hip flexor muscles are called upon to bend at the hips. Several muscles of the pelvis and thigh contribute to hip flexion, but those primarily involved are the psoas major and iliacus (often referred to collectively as the iliopsoas), with assistance from the rectus femoris. Also involved are the abdominal and erector spinae (lower back) muscles. Although they don't contribute to hip flexion, they serve to keep the upper torso erect and the spine in place.

Except for abdominal exercises, all other movements that require bending at the midsection should be done from the hips. Classic examples are squats and deadlifts, but even upper-body exercises like bent-over rows, triceps kickbacks and some rear-deltoid movements require bending that must come from the hips.

The Way of the Waist

Abdominal movements are the prime hip flexor, reduce its involvement during abdominal movements to emphasize contraction of the rectus abdominis. To accomplish this, bend your knees or position the thighs almost perpendicular (90 degrees) to the lower torso during upper-abdominal exercises.

'Except for abdominal exercises, all other movements that require bending at the midsection should be done from the hips.'

exception to the rule; here, bending at the waist is not only encouraged but required. Bending at the waist implies spinal flexion, or forward bending of the spine. This is usually acceptable in an unloaded (lying, hanging or inverted) position but is never recommended in a loaded (body upright, weights overhead) position. Even without weights, your head and upper torso provide enough weight to place significant force upon the vertebral discs of the lower back during spinal flexion. Such forces can cause immediate injury or lead to chronic back problems over time.

The primary muscles responsible for spinal flexion are the rectus abdominis and iliopsoas. Since the iliopsoas is also a

The range of motion for spinal flexion is very small, as evidenced by the small movement used to perform the abdominal crunch. To properly execute spinal flexion, think of bringing your ribcage and your pelvis (hips) together. To ensure complete abdominal contraction and lower-ab involvement, also rotate your pelvis backward by flattening your lower back at the same time.

24

EXHALE AFTER EXERTION

A: Yes. Breathing is a critical component of successful training, though it rarely gets much attention. To make matters worse, the little information that gets circulated is often incorrect. It's important to understand that breathing is more than a means to exchange oxygen and carbon dioxide — it's the foundation for safe and productive training.

Consider what you do when you're trying to relax. Most likely you take a deep breath, then exhale. So why would you exhale during a lift, at the very moment you're exerting maximal force? Probably because that's what you were taught — to exhale as the weight is lifted. But, in fact, this is only partially true. You should exhale only after you've passed the point of peak exertion; otherwise you put your body in a vulnerable position, increasing your risk of injury.

Holding your breath during a lift increases intra-abdominal pressure, which holds your spine in place and makes your entire midsection more stable. It's like having a built-in lifting belt, activated every time you hold your breath. "Don't limit it only to intra-abdominal [pressure]; it's also intra-thoracic," states Michael Yessis, PhD, president of Sports Training Inc. in Escondido, California. "It's the total torso. The breath-holding, in essence, stabilizes the whole torso, from the hips to the head. And here's where the safety factor comes in."

"When you hold your breath, it stabilizes the torso — it makes it rigid. When it's rigid, you have a stable core against which the muscles can effectively contract. But if you have a weak, loose core, then you don't have a firm base against which the muscles are able to pull. So you have both ends of the muscles in motion, and that can lead to injury."

The increased torso stability achieved from breath-holding translates into improved leverage and the ability to generate more force. Yessis explains: "When you hold your breath, you're a lot stronger. The Russians have done studies on this where they estimated people to be a good 20% or more stronger when they hold their breath." In short, holding your breath through the sticking point of an exercise lets

you train heavier, thereby building greater strength and muscle mass.

Concerned about the increased blood pressure associated with breath-holding and resistance training? Keep in mind that the breath is held only for a brief period (maybe 3–5

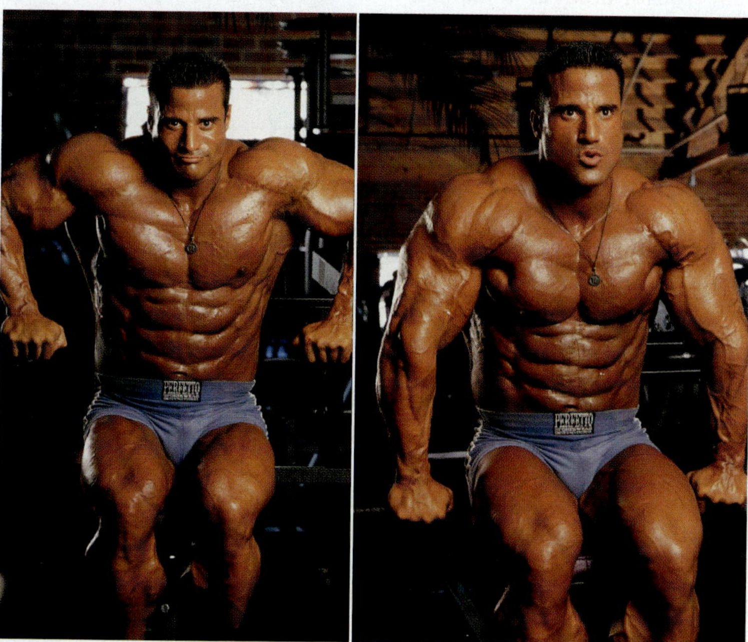

Exhaling during the right moment allows you to generate more force.

seconds) and is then forcefully exhaled. You'll still be in the concentric (lifting) phase when you exhale, but beyond the point of maximal exertion. This practice is safe for healthy individuals, but inadvisable for those with cardiovascular conditions, who probably shouldn't be lifting

heavy weights anyway. (Check with your physician first.)

In addition, the breaths you take and hold should not be extreme but rather just slightly more than normal. Yessis tells his clients, "Inhale more than what you're used to, but not maximally."

Another benefit of breath-holding is increased strength of the respiratory muscles. "Improving the strength of your respiratory muscles is another part of the total fitness equation," Yessis adds. "The respiratory and cardiovascular systems are tied in, so here's another way of improving both systems and increasing performance."

If you're still not convinced, observe your own breathing habits the next time you're at the gym. Odds are you already hold your breath during maximal exertion. Your body knows what's best for you, and will automatically breath-hold as a natural reflex to exertion. Continue to follow these simple guidelines and you'll breath some life into your training program!

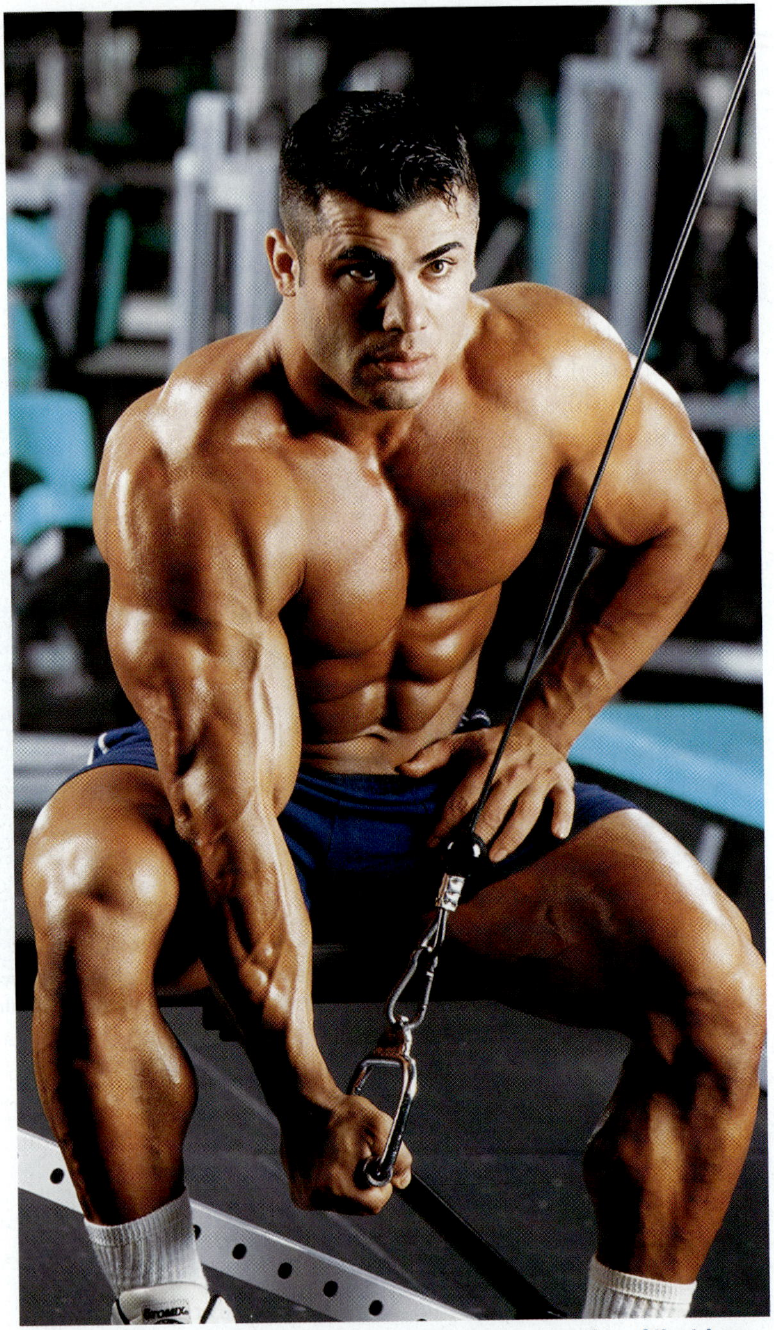

25

LOCK OUT WITH CARE

I've read where some bodybuilders say to lock out on particular movements, but other times I hear that locking out is bad for your joints. Which is it?

A: Locking out describes when you take an exercise to full extension of a joint, typically a knee or elbow. Certain contraindications and conditions make joint lockout a dangerous practice, but most

Many bodybuilders lock out the elbow to get peak contraction of the triceps.

bodybuilders can benefit from a program that includes it.

If you were to take a poll asking bodybuilders their opinion on locking out, some would agree that it's acceptable with triceps movements (elbow joint), but most would advise against doing so with the knee joint. When asked to elaborate, they might explain that locking out places undue stress on the knee, possibly leading to injury. Yet what you sacrifice when you don't lock out is the end of the range of motion and an important training principle: peak contraction.

Let's back up for a moment to make one distinction clear: There's a fine line between safe and unsafe lockout, and the variables that separate one from the other are speed and force. Movements performed to lockout in a slow, controlled fashion are typically considered safe. Explosive, ballistic or heavy movements that result in lockout can be dangerous because of the high forces and the risk of hyperextension — the exten-

sion of a joint beyond its normal limits, often resulting in damage to the connective tissue (tendons and ligaments) or the joint itself.

Some exercises — plyometrics, for example — are designed to be executed quickly and explosively, and must be done so to be effective. But these movements rarely involve weights that exceed bodyweight, and any weight used is typically released before the joint reaches lockout. So even though the movements incorporate high speeds, the lighter weights limit the forces applied to the joint.

Another risk for injury stems from movements performed with excessive weight, like heavy squats or french presses. If such movements are performed to the point of forceful lockout, the momentum and forces generated can easily override the body's mechanisms to stop the weight. If this happens, the possibility of hyperextension and subsequent injury is greatly increased.

If you have a pre-existing con-

dition that involves injury, degeneration or instability of the elbow or knee joints, it goes without saying that lockout should be used sparingly and with light weights and slow movements only. In addition, any movements that cause pain or undue discomfort in these joints should be performed with caution, especially when nearing the point of full extension.

Even if your joints are healthy, always take care when taking an exercise to the point of lockout. Use slow and controlled movements, but if speed is required, reduce the resistance to lessen the forces applied to the joint. Training smart will allow most bodybuilders to incorporate lockout in their workouts, thereby maximizing contraction, range of motion and muscle stimulation.

'**Explosive movements that result in lockout can be dangerous because of the risk of hyperextension.**'

26

ALL IN THE GRIP

Does the training emphasis of the seated row change significantly when I switch from a narrow grip to a wide one?

A: Changing your grip width when doing seated rows causes a corresponding change in elbow position that, although slight, is enough to alter muscle involvement and the angle of stress placed on each muscle.

Remember when you first started training? No matter what you did, muscle gain seemed almost effortless. Whether you knew it or not, most of the gains were a result of your muscles and nerves learning to work together to perform movements efficiently. But once they learned the movements and adapted to the resistance, your gains began to taper.

That's why you need to continually challenge your muscles by changing the resistance and exercise angles you use. This forces your nervous system to recruit muscle fibers differently, leading to adaptation and growth. Although that growth is unlikely to be as significant as when you first started, by altering your training, you'll minimize the plateaus. Continued growth is the key to successful bodybuilding, and subtle changes in the

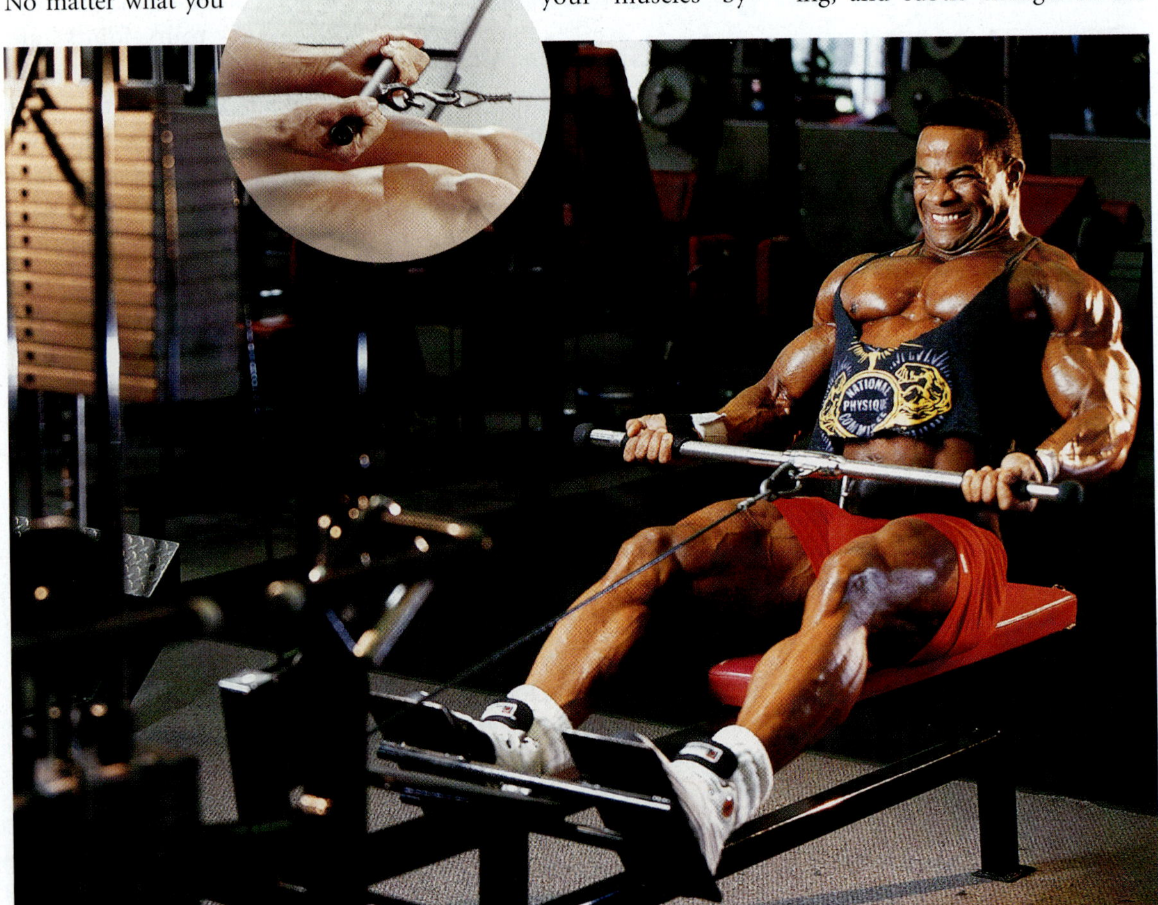

You should alternate between wide and narrow grips on seated rows to stimulate maximum muscle fiber recruitment.

way you train go a long way toward making it happen.

Narrow Grip

When you use a narrow grip, your elbows are at shoulder width and move straight back, resulting in shoulder extension — backward movement of the upper arm in the vertical plane. Shoulder extension involves the muscles of the upper back and shoulder, including the latissimus dorsi (lats), teres major (shoulder blade region) and the rear head of the deltoid (shoulder).

When the elbows cross the midpoint of the body during their pulling movement, the shoulder blades rotate down and in. These movements require contraction of the major and minor rhomboids, as well as the middle trapezius muscles. All three are located in the middle portion of the upper back.

Wide Grip

A wide grip, especially overhand, forces the elbows out, leading to shoulder extension in a plane that's more horizontal than vertical. The rear delts and teres minor are more involved, and shoulder blade movement shifts from down to in. This inward movement (adduction) of the shoulder blades is the sole purpose of the middle trap, so using the wide grip is a great way to

develop this potentially massive portion of your back.

Exercise Mechanics

Regardless of the grip width you use, you'll perform the seated row nearly the same. Your knees should be slightly bent and your upper torso erect, with perhaps a slightly exaggerated arch in your back. Don't lean forward or backward, which merely involves the lower back (for which this exercise is not designed). Concentrate on bringing your elbows down and back, trying to touch your shoulder blades together.

With the close grip, keep your elbows in close to your body. A neutral grip in which your palms face each other can help you do this. Conversely, with the wide grip, keep your elbows out and away.

By altering your favorite exercises regularly, in even slight ways such as this, you'll be able to stimulate your muscles on an ongoing basis and avoid the dreaded plateau.

27

RED-FLAG EXERCISES

Over the years, I've seen certain exercises pop up repeatedly in the pros' routines, then I turn around and read other articles explaining the hazards of those exercises. I'm thinking specifically of the behind-the-neck press. I've read that this exercise should be avoided because it isn't as natural as the seated or standing military press, and that it puts strain on different areas of the body that can lead to injury. What's the deal?

A: When people talk about dangerous exercises, they're really talking about dangerous technique. If you take your body through a natural movement, with or without resistance, you shouldn't incur any sort of injury. A natural movement, for example, is bending your elbow, something you can certainly do without injury. However, if you bend your elbow in such a way that stress is

'Injuries typically occur for one or more of these reasons: Using too much weight too soon, using poor technique and overtraining.'

being applied to it from the side, so that you're basically fighting the natural arc of the movement, then that's a different story. This stress from the side places strain on virtually all the relevant connective tissues, and if this occurs long enough or with enough severity, you'll be injured.

The same principle holds true for the behind-the-neck press. This movement is certainly natural, but if you bring the bar down low enough, you end up placing an inordinate amount of strain on the tendons and ligaments of your shoulders. If the strain is severe enough, you can injure yourself. How severe is too severe? Person A might be able to bring the bar down as low as possible and never suffer any problems. Person B might do it only once before having to visit the doctor.

It's impossible to say definitively what your body can take during specific exercises without getting injured. Such answers are hard to come by because individual genetics plays a fundamental role. However, everyone who trains should realize that injuries typically occur for one or more of these reasons: Using too much weight too soon, using poor technique and overtraining.

If you progress slowly and don't add excessive poundage before you're conditioned enough to do so, you should be fine. If you pay particularly close attention to proper technique, you can dramatically decrease the probability of getting injured. Lastly, you can prevent injuries by allowing yourself a sufficient amount of rest (say, 72 hours) before hitting the same bodypart again. To take it a step further, don't blast your muscles week in and week out without a break. Hit 'em hard for about three weeks and then back off for a week, during which you reduce your sets, reps and poundage by 30%–40%. Then work your way back up to your previous weight and try to surpass it before taking another short break.

All in all, genetics and poor attention to certain training variables are more likely to cause injury rather than partic-

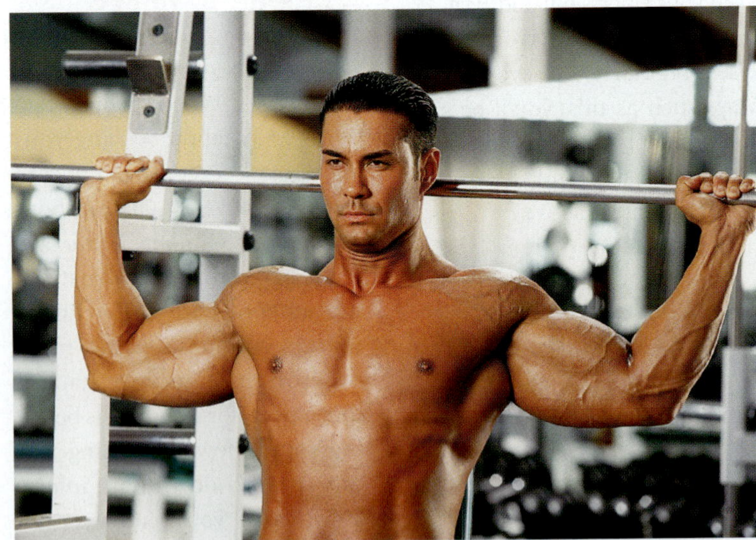

Avoid bringing the bar down too low when doing a behind-the-neck press.

ular exercises. By adopting a smart approach to training, you should be able to avoid injuries altogether.

28

POSITIVE VS. NEGATIVE

What's the difference between a concentric contraction and an eccentric one? Which is more important for building muscle?

A: Bodybuilding movements consist of reps, and each one includes both a concentric and an eccentric contraction, separated by a brief pause. The phases move resistance in opposite directions, but both contribute toward a common goal — muscle development!

A concentric contraction is a movement in which the muscle shortens as it contracts, demonstrated by the biceps muscle in the upward motion of a biceps curl. When the direction is reversed and the weight is lowered, the biceps muscle remains con-

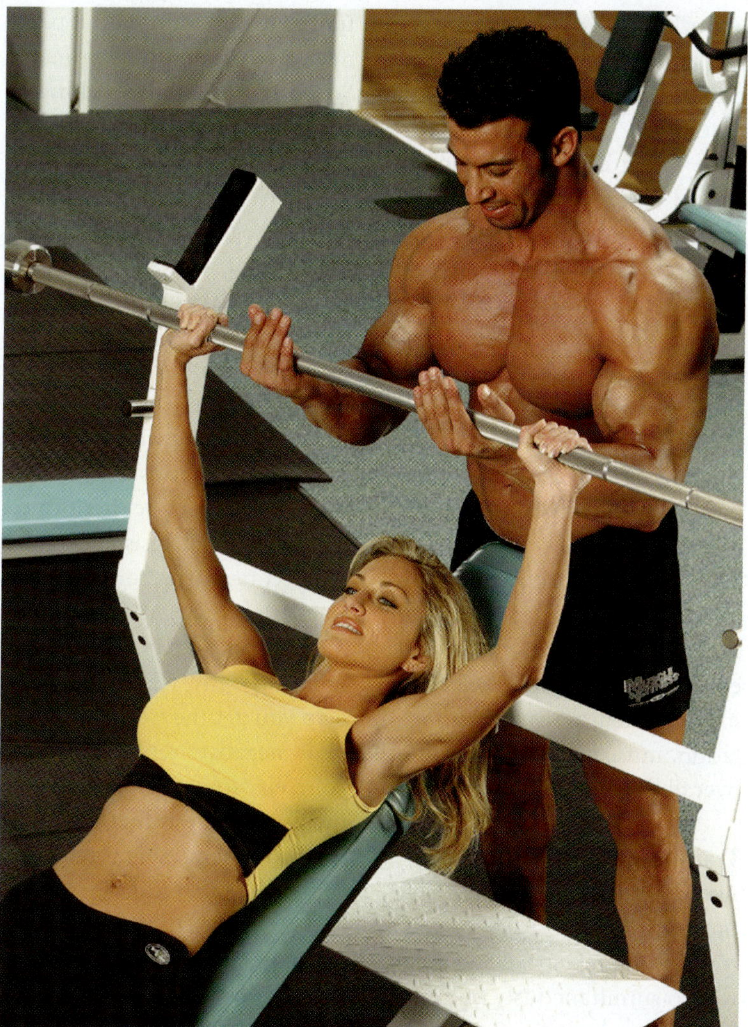

For negatives, lower the weight slowly and have your partner help you lift it up.

tracted, but switches to an eccentric contraction: a movement in which the muscle lengthens during contraction.

The concentric contraction is usually the lifting portion of an exercise, while the eccentric contraction is the segment that

returns the weight to the starting position. Unfortunately, some bodybuilders still think of the concentric phase as the "muscle-building" portion, and the eccentric phase as a mere transition back to the concentric phase.

Both phases of contraction are important for complete muscle development. You can't ignore the eccentric component of an exercise (doing so would likely send weights crashing to the floor), but lack of attention may limit your growth potential. By focusing equally on the eccentric and concentric contractions, constant tension is maintained throughout the movement, causing increased muscle fatigue. Additionally, neural adaptations that take place for each type of contraction are specific to that contraction. Targeting both concentric and eccentric contractions will elicit maximal neuromuscular stimulation, muscle-fiber fatigue and overall development.

Training Eccentrically

Avoiding overly explosive movements and instead controlling the rep speed is a great way to simultaneously train the

'Eccentric movements can be performed with a greater resistance than their concentric counterparts.'

concentric and eccentric phases. To actively train the eccentric phase, however, you're bet-

ter off if you train with a partner or with special equipment. Some gyms have isokinetic equipment that allows specific eccentric training; otherwise, you can train eccentrically by doing negatives on a Smith machine or with a partner (the term negative simply refers to the negative or eccentric phase of a movement).

Start with the weight in the "up" position, slowly lowering it for 3–5 seconds. Eccentric movements can be performed with a greater resistance than their concentric counterparts, so choose a weight that's about 20% heavier than you would normally lift. Have a spotter help you get the weight up after each negative rep — or spot yourself for one-arm movements. Go easy at first, as eccentric movements are more stressful on the muscle fibers and incur more damage. Subsequently, increased muscle soreness can be expected, espe-

cially during the first few weeks.

Certainly, quick movements and speed work have a place in

training, but bodybuilders desiring mass should stick to slow, controlled movements that concentrate on utilizing every muscle fiber. Give the eccentric movements equal time and consideration when you're in the gym, and you'll find that not only are more muscle fibers incorporated, but they're exhausted to a greater extent. With adequate rest and nutrition, gains in muscle mass are sure to follow.

29

SPEED & GAINS

I'd like to know about the different speeds for lifting weights. Which is most effective — slow, medium or fast?

A: This is an important and complicated topic. The speed of your reps is important because of the impact on performance and complicated because of the way the research is conducted. Steven Fleck, PhD, CSCS, and William Kraemer, PhD, CSCS, probably put it best: ". . . No conclusive answer has emerged."[1] But as we sift through the research, we'd have to conclude that you could expect greater gains in strength and size if you were to train explosively and that the effort you put forth is probably more important than speed per se.

Because research methods require consistent, controllable and measurable conditions, studies on rep speed tend to use isokinetic devices. These machines allow researchers to select a specific movement speed that's maintained throughout the range of motion, which in turn allows for direct comparisons from subject to subject; this type of consistency is hard to maintain with dumbbells and barbells. Now, a study conducted by Michelle Lacerte, et al, from the University of Washington, Seattle, found positive and negative slow contractions (60 degrees per second) to be superior in terms of peak torque (strength about a joint) to faster

'You could expect greater gains if you were to train explosively and the effort you put forth is probably more important than speed.'

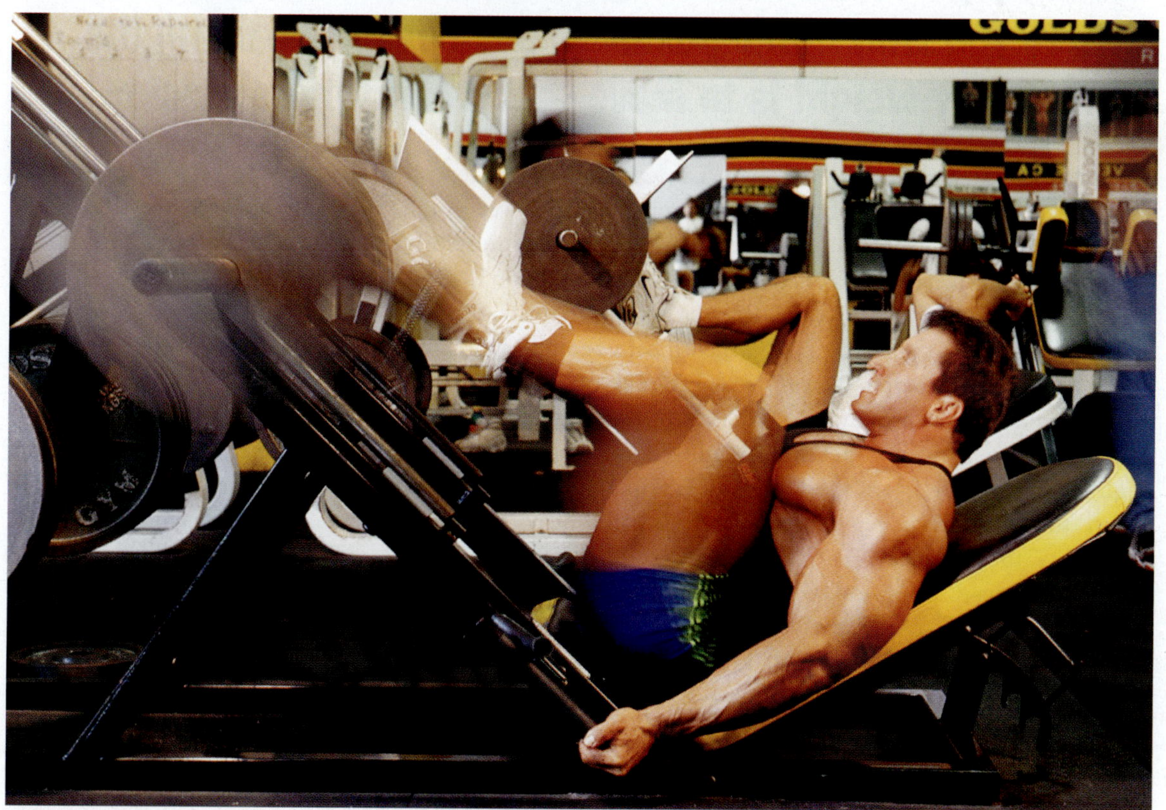

For best results from a movement, lift heavy weights as quickly as possible. This places greater demand on your muscles.

ones (180 degrees per second).[2]

Similar results were found by E.F. Coyle, et al,[3] where the slower-speed group improved peak torque significantly more than the fast group (by 8%). A study out of the Department of Exercise Physiology at Rigshospitalet University Hospital, Copenhagen, Denmark, examined velocities of 30, 120 and 240 degrees per second during (one-second) squat speed, scientists found that the fast-squatting group increased strength more than the slow-squatting group.[5]

Based on the research, our advice is to lift heavy weight (a rep range of 3–8) as quickly as possible. Here's why: First, consider that the more difficult the lift or the more effort it takes to complete a lift, the more gains to first break down before they can rebuild to the next level. A sufficient degree of muscle breakdown can't be achieved unless you increase the intensity of your work by moving progressively heavier weights and moving those weights quickly.

Fourth, don't overlook the importance of the negative. Though it appears you don't need to be too concerned with

'The way you can make things harder in the weight room (where you won't find isokinetic devices) while using the same heavy weight is to move that weight more quickly.'

isokinetic leg extensions and leg curls. A close look at the negative part of the lift showed gains at all speeds, irrespective of training speed.[4]

At first glance, then, you'd think that slow is better. Not really. You see, in an isokinetic machine, a slower speed requires greater resistance or effort to complete a rep. So basically the subjects got stronger because they worked harder. Now, with heavy barbells and dumbbells (80% or more of your one-rep max), moving the weight more quickly through the range of motion is more demanding. By looking at slow (two-second) and fast you can expect in the strength department. Since slower isokinetic contractions are more difficult to execute, you'll find greater results in peak torque, which most equate to increased strength. The only way you can make things harder in the weight room (where you won't find isokinetic devices) while using the same heavy weight is to move that weight more quickly. Second, since moving weight more quickly places a greater demand on your muscles and nervous system, you should also experience greater gains in size.

Third, a rather well-established fact is that muscles need rep speed here, maintaining a reasonable speed to control the weight seems smart.

How quick is quick enough? In terms of barbells, dumbbells and typical machines, the actual time it takes to move a weight may not be as important as the degree of effort you put forth. If your max bench is 300 pounds, you'd better explode and move it as fast as possible, otherwise the bar will stay on your chest. But with less weight, you have a choice in speed. The demand on your muscle fibers and nervous system would be greater with greater speed, so look at using predominantly quick and explosive reps for greater gains.

30

SPOTTING A GOOD WORKOUT

My job requires that I travel extensively, so I typically find myself training alone. Even when others are present, I'm not comfortable asking a total stranger for a spot. What can I do to get the most out of my workouts without a spotter?

A: Filling the void left by the absence of a good training partner, especially the role he or she plays as a spotter, is difficult. But with some standard equipment and a little resourcefulness, you can safely train alone without sacrificing the benefits of a spotter. Here are a few ideas to consider.

The Smith Machine

The Smith machine is the solo lifter's best friend. Essentially, this free-weight apparatus allows barbell movement in a vertical plane only. The guides can limit the freedom of motion slightly, but that's a small tradeoff for the ability to lock the bar's movement with a twist of your wrist. A variety of movements can be performed on the Smith machine, and with the built-in safety hooks, you don't have to worry about failing on the last rep. So go ahead, lift as heavy as you like, or load it up and do some heavy reps. You'll find the Smith machine to be quite ver-

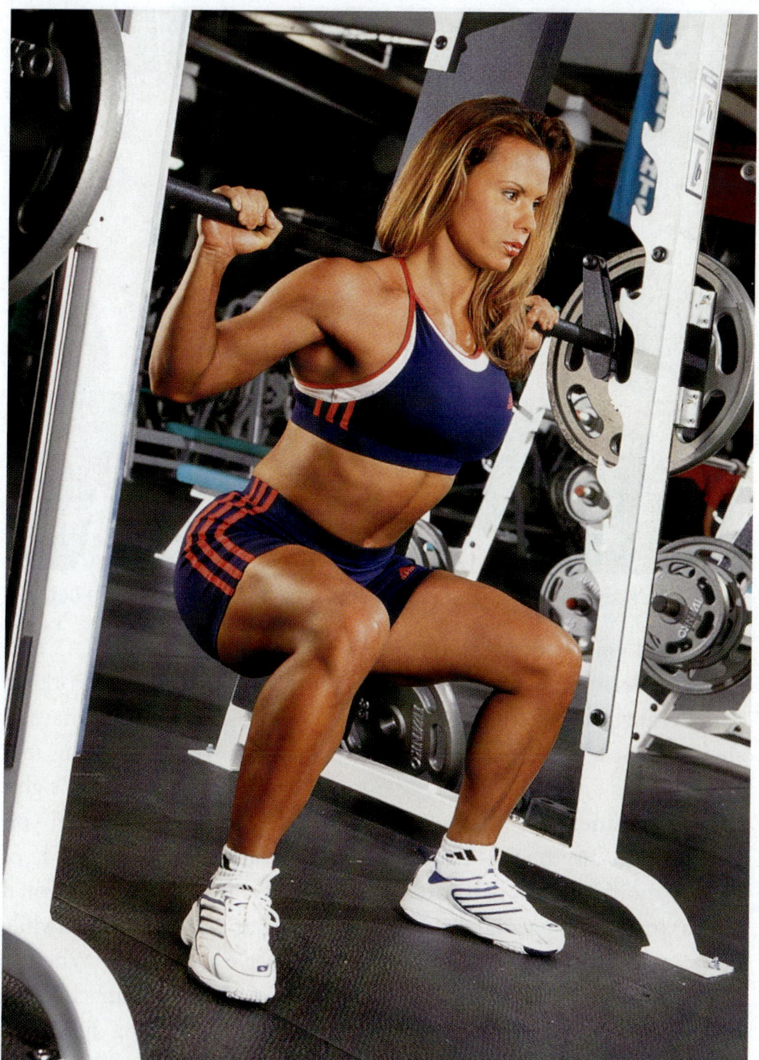

A Smith machine is a safe and effective way to perform squats without a spotter.

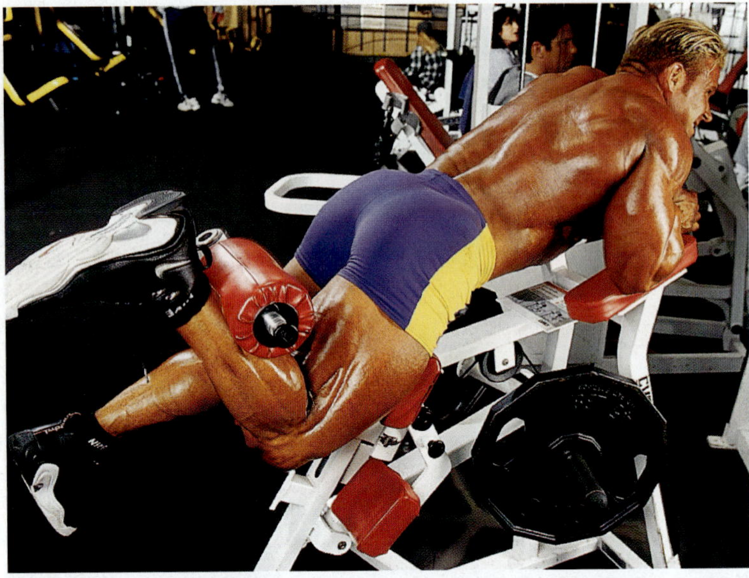

Don't have a spotter? Unilateral movements on a machine are a safe bet.

satile, and you'll never catch its eyes wandering when you suddenly realize you need immediate assistance.

Other Machines

Free weights are the first choice of any bodybuilder dedicated to maximizing muscular development, but machines do have a time and place. One of those times is when you feel the need to lift heavy but don't have a spotter. Most new equipment is well designed and will effectively stimulate the target muscle. Trying new machines will add variety to your workouts and can also stress the muscle in a slightly different way than it's accustomed to.

Unilateral Movements

Before giving up on a workout just because you don't have a spotter, consider spotting for yourself. Yeah, you read it right. Think about any movement you perform unilaterally (one side of the body at a time) and you'll realize that one limb is free while the other is working. Whether you're using a cable, machine or dumbbell, the resting limb can assist when the other side reaches the point of muscular failure.

Other Techniques

Maybe you're stuck in one of those hotels that has only an old Universal Gym or just a few assorted dumbbells. No point in working out if you can't lift heavy, right? Wrong. Now's the perfect time to change things up a bit and do something your muscles won't expect. Why not use less resistance and add more reps? Give yourself a good endurance workout, maybe even do a circuit that hits all the major muscle groups. What about doing some cardio? We all need it, and most places at the very least have a pool and/or stairs.

Whatever situation you find yourself in, remember that being without a spotter isn't a valid excuse for skipping a workout. Use some imagination with the equipment you have, and you'll discover ways to add zest to your training routine.

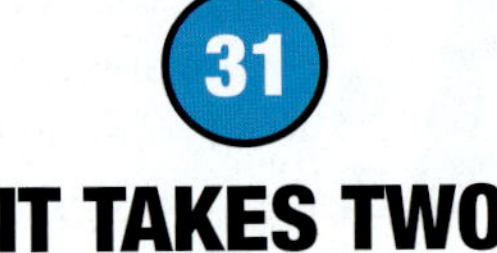

IT TAKES TWO

I've been training solo for a couple of years, but sometimes skip workouts and seem to lack motivation to train. Do you think having a training partner will make a big difference, and what should I be

looking for in this individual?

A: Bodybuilding may be an individual sport, but nobody makes it to any place of success without the help of others. Think of the countless early mornings, the forced reps, the diets, the pats on the back, the kicks in the butt, and the words of encouragement spoken not to impress but rather to push you to greater gains. Henry Ford once said, "My best friend is the one who brings out the best in me." For the training partner, that means using the right intensity, the right motivation, and having the knowledge to be safe and effective to help fulfill your partner's training goals and dreams.

A good training partner can't be just anyone. He or she has to be:

Someone Who Knows How to Spot

We've all been there: The enormity of weight on the bench has drawn a crowd. All have postponed their next set to watch the strongman display. He gets a liftoff and barely completes a rep. The spotter, however, does a full set of bent-over rows to get his partner to 10 reps — all the while yelling, "It's all you, dude, it's aaaaaall (grunt) you."

Partners who help too much are a common sight, but the risks — including diminished gains as well as injury to both people — definitely outweigh any benefits. Simply put, your partner needs to know when and how much to spot.

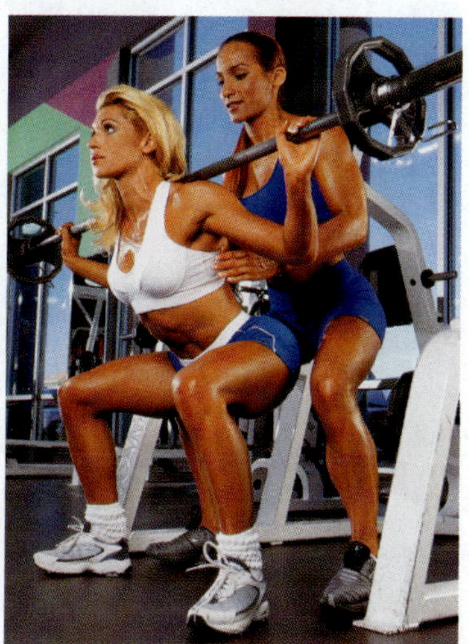

A good workout partner should help keep her partner moving with the weight.

The key is constant motion, with as much work as possible coming from the lifter. Clichéd as it may sound, safety and proper spotting technique really do come first, and a major focus of any partner should be the well-being of his counterpart. Knowing when and how to keep your partner moving with the weight, knowing when your partner has bitten off more than he can chew, and understanding form well enough to correct improper technique are all necessary qualities.

Someone Who Is Reliable

Chances are, every bodybuilder you ask would agree that consistency and reliability are the keys to being a good training partner. If the clock strikes the training hour and you're a no-show, it diminishes and compromises the integrity of your training-partner relationship.

Someone Who Is Attentive

A partner should be more than just attentive; he should work the weight with you every step of the way. The camaraderie between partners should be evident in the ability of each to block out distractions and concentrate on the set.

Someone Who Can Communicate to Meet on Common Ground

You've probably trained with

'Consistency and reliability are the keys to being a good training partner.'

someone who thinks he needs to say something during every rep of every set on every exercise. (They're usually the ones who can't keep quiet between sets, either.) Though his intentions are good, the results can be distracting and counterproductive. Saying the right things at the right times helps workout partners get the best out of each other.

As in any other relationship, communication between training partners is vital. They might have different viewpoints on the best way to perform a particular exercise or disagree on the number of sets and reps to best maximize growth, but such differences can be used as a springboard to further gains. Partners can learn from each other's mistakes and intertwine theories. The partner's job is to make sure that whatever form or tactic his partner chooses, he's doing it to the best of his ability.

Someone Who Is Willing to Sacrifice

Regardless of ability level, the person you want assistance from in the gym is the one willing to commit to helping you reach your goals, and vice versa.

And Finally, Someone Who Is Motivating

A great training partner is someone who can play the the other picks him up.

Everyone has bad days, and your training partner should be there to get you back on track. He needs to know how to push your buttons and say the things you need to hear to get your adrenalin pumping and your mind focused on the workout.

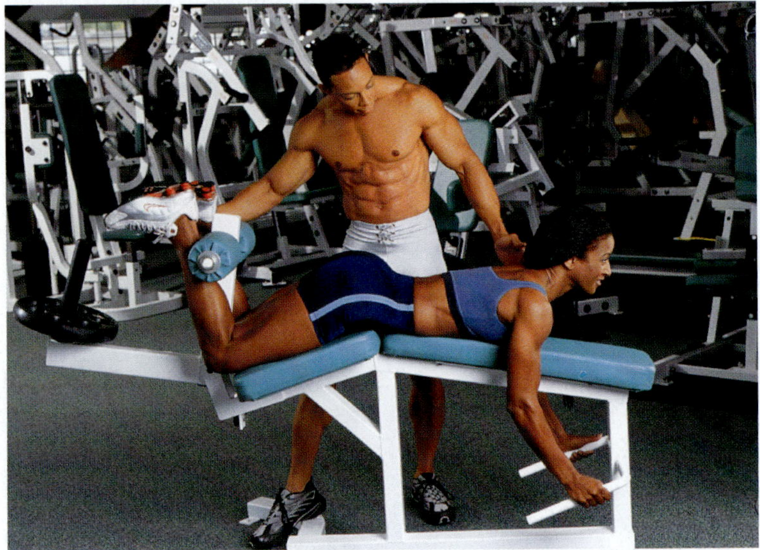

The majority of the work should come from the lifter, not his or her training partner.

heavy when you aren't in the mood for a great workout. The ideal training partnership goes both ways: When one is down, This may be the most important characteristic separating the good training partner from the great one. ■

References

1. Fleck, S., Kraemer, W. Designing resistance training programs. Champaign, IL: Human Kinetics, 1997.

2. Lacerte, M., deLateur, B.J., Alquist, A.D., Questad, K.A. Concentric versus combined concentric-eccentric isokinetic training programs: effect on peak torque of human quadriceps femoris muscle. Archives of Physical Medicine and Rehabilitation 73(11):1,059–1,062, 1992.

3. Coyle, E.F., Feiring, D.C., Rotkis, T.C., et al. Specificity of power improvements through slow and fast isokinetic training. Journal of Applied Physiology 51(6):1,437–1,442, 1981.

4. Aagaard, P., Simonsen, E.B., Trolle, M., et al. Specificity of training velocity and training load on gains in isokinetic knee joint strength. Acta Physiologica Scandinavia 156(2):123–129, 1996.

5. Morrissey, M.C., Harman, E.A., Frykman, P.N., Han, K.H. Early phase differential effects of slow and fast barbell squat training. American Journal of Sports Medicine 26(2):221–230, 1998.

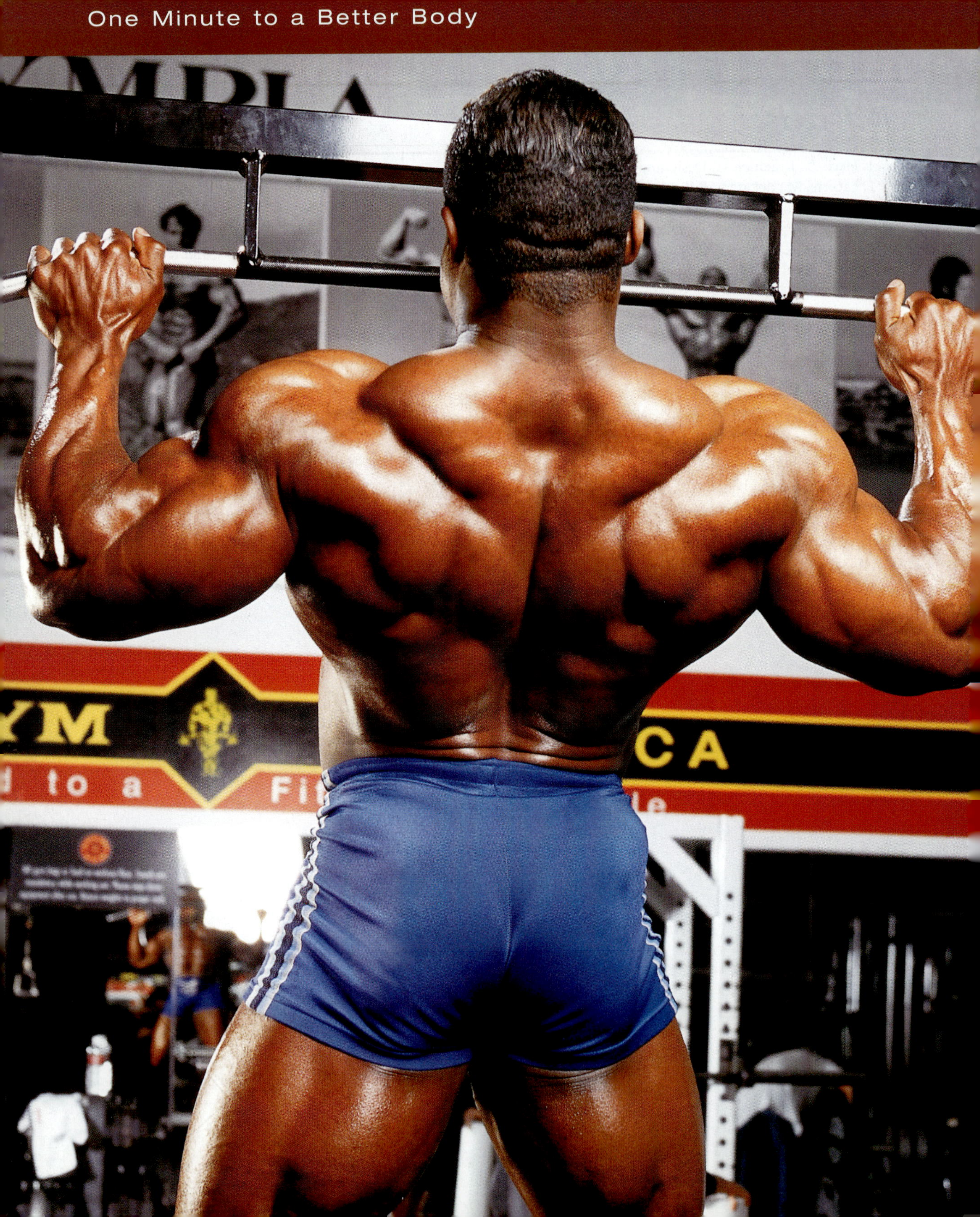

GREAT GUNS AND A SIX-PACK

Exercise techniques and tips for a hard upper body

If you're setting your sights on 19-inch arms and a six-pack, you're not alone. From delts to obliques, it seems that the upper body gets the most attention on the beach, and in the bedroom. There are countless ways to train your upper body, but some strategies work better than others. And that's the point of this section: identifying the optimal ways to train your abs, arms, shoulders, chest and back. Before we get started with the questions and answers, here's a brief overview of the parts we'll be covering.

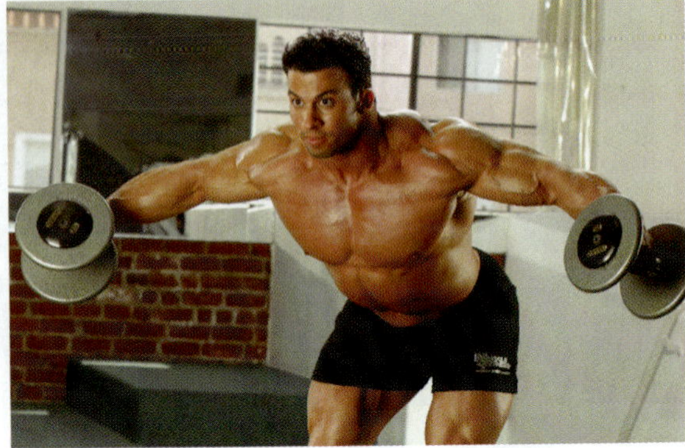

Admirable Midsection

The muscle group most commonly referred to as the abs is composed of four separate muscles — the rectus abdominis, the internal and external obliques, and the transverse abdominis. Although the rectus abdominis is a single muscle, you can work it from different angles to better target particular areas. Though you can never truly isolate the upper-ab region from the lower, the answer to question 33 will tell you how to maximize stress on one area over the other.

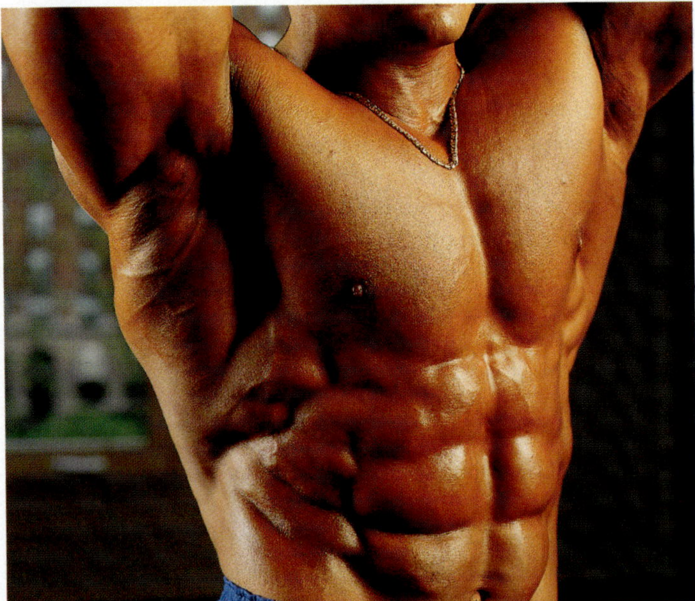

Bigger Back

If you want wings of muscle to contribute to a V-shape, you need to work your lats. In this section, you'll learn how to incorporate a handful of basic lat exercises into an unlimited number of movements, simply by making minor modifications. For example, did you know that your grip affects which part of the lats is stressed in pull-downs? Or that leaning forward when performing a row shifts the emphasis to the lower back — something you probably don't want. Find out why on page 92 .

Better Bi's

Sleeve-busting bi's can be achieved by inducing maximum muscle contraction. This doesn't mean you have to max out every workout or go to failure on every set, but it does mean you must overload your arms just enough to make them grow. The smartest approach to increasing arm size is to periodically change the weight as well as the number of sets and reps you do in a calculated way (called periodization). For example, start off with relatively light weights for a number of sets, then progress to gradually reduce volume (sets and reps) and increase intensity (weight, or RM). Again, the goal of periodizing your arm training is to progressively overload your arm muscles while avoiding overtraining. If you just can't wait to find out how to get the "ball effect" pros like Ronnie Coleman sport, flip to page 95. Otherwise, let's move on to the chest.

Chest Above the Rest

The muscle we tend to refer to when discussing the chest is named pectoralis major, hence the nickname "pecs." Working along with these is the smaller pectoralis minor, which lies underneath and is trained in conjunction with its larger counterpart. You should always train the pecs fresh and first: fresh, as in once every 5-7 days; first, as in before any other muscle group you pair with it on a given training day. There are two major types of chest movements: presses and flyes. Presses are multijoint movements, so start with them as you can typically go fairly heavy, and follow with isolation exercises like flyes. Speaking of flyes, are you performing them correctly? Find out on page 105.

Bolder Shoulders

Whether you're a man or a woman, well-defined shoulders mark you as part of the bodybuilding clan. The delts include the front (anterior) delt, middle (side) delt and rear

(posterior) delt. You need to train each area to maximize shoulder size and strength. Begin with a compound, or multijoint, movement since these involve multiple heads. Be sure to include single-joint exercises to target each of the three heads of the delt. While every bodybuilder has his or her own preference as to the order in which to do isolation exercises, you should not follow the same order for too long or you risk underdeveloping the last muscle group you trained in your routine. You can avoid this by rotating the delt heads: training

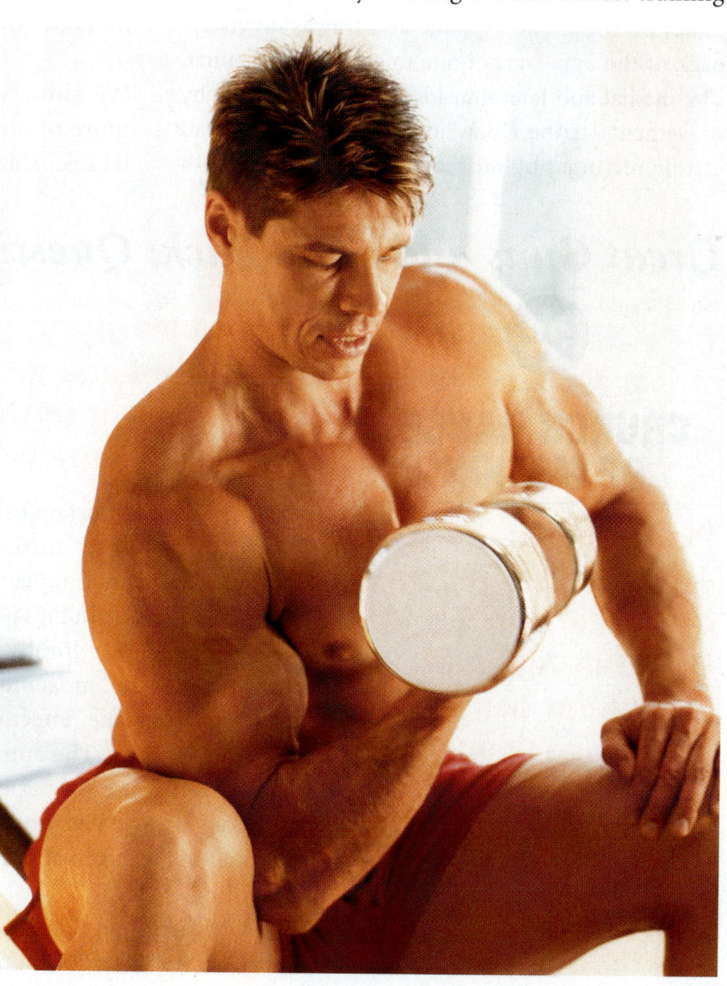

the front first in one workout, the rear first the next, and so on.

Tightening Those Tri's

Once you understand the anatomy of the triceps brachii, you'll realize why you can't simply perform pressdowns and dips until the cows come home and expect to achieve complete triceps development. Whereas the medial and lateral heads originate on the upper-arm bone and attach on the ulna — one of the forearm bones — the long head originates on the shoulder blade and travels down the back of the upper-arm bone to attach on the ulna. The medial and lateral heads are recruited only by movements at the elbow joint, and the long head can be recruited by movements occurring at both

'Performing an exercise through its full range of motion leads to fuller muscle development.'

the elbow and shoulder joints. What this means is that to fully stretch the long head of the triceps, you must raise your upper arms overhead, as you do during overhead extensions. On page 113 you'll find out how to target other parts of the triceps.

We know you're anxious to get the answers to more of our most frequently asked questions, so let's get started.

Great Guns and a Six-Pack: Questions and Answers

32

CRUNCH RANGE OF MOTION

I've heard that exercises should be executed through their full range of motion for complete muscle development. Does this concept apply to the abdominal crunch? If so, how high should I go up, and should I let my shoulders come all the way down to the floor between reps?

A: It is important to do crunches through their full range of motion, but it's possible to exceed the limits on either end of the movement, detracting from the effectiveness of the exercise. The appropriate range of motion permits continuous muscle tension — a vital tool for successful abdominal training.

Performing an exercise through its full range of motion leads to fuller muscle development by ensuring the fibers are stimulated at every possible point through the movement. Limiting the range of motion merely limits muscle involvement and stimulation.

Movement about most joints is distinct with relatively concrete end limits. Such is not the case with the abdominals, particularly the rectus abdominis — the most visible abdominal muscle and primary target of ab training. Unless you know where to stop on either end, your ab training may be highly inefficient and incorporate unwanted muscles.

At the top of the movement, the end of concentric contraction, your upper body should be at about 30 degrees to the floor. Range of motion for the rectus abdominis is quite small, so movement beyond 30 degrees brings into play other muscles, namely the hip flexors. Contraction should be thought of as shortening the space between the ribcage and pelvis (hips). Think of touching your lower ribs to your hips as you concentrate on maximally compressing (shortening) your abdominals. Little or no movement is desired at the hips, upper back and neck.

On the way down, stop just short of your shoulders touching the floor. Once your shoulders hit the floor, abdominal tension is released, allowing the muscles to relax. The abdominals are a resilient muscle group, accustomed to repeated contraction throughout the day. To make them grow, you have to fatigue them much more than they're used to. They also recover quickly,

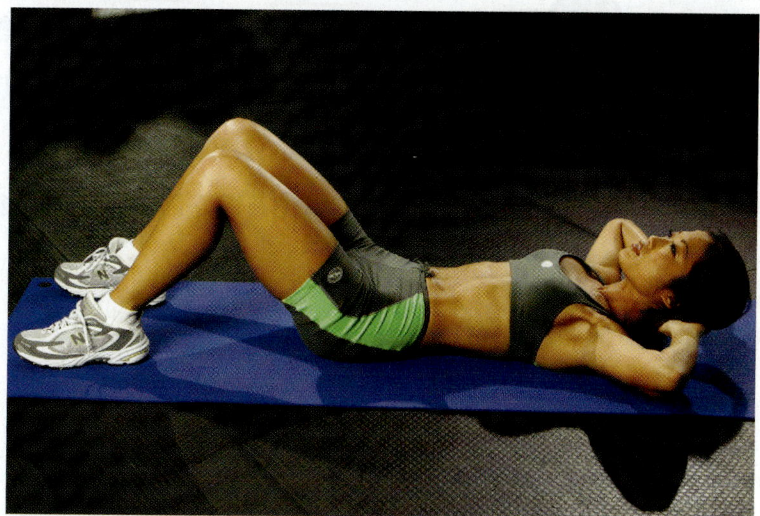

During a crunch, think of shortening the space between your ribcage and hips.

making it extremely difficult to exhaust them if they're allowed to rest even briefly between reps.

Those with back problems or who experience back pain during the crunch movement may have to return completely to the floor to rest the spinal erectors. The erectors are the complementary muscles of the lower back that, together with the abdominals, form a natural "belt" of muscle around the waist necessary for torso stability. The erectors are in a state of contraction during the descent phase of the crunch, which may aggravate the lower back of some individuals. If back pain persists, choose another abdominal exercise that permits pain-free execution or consult a health-care professional.

Most of the time, more is better, but not in the case of the crunch. Keep the range of motion short and within the functional limits of the rectus abdominis. Strive for continuous tension and slow, controlled movements of maximal effort and contraction.

'The abdominals are a resilient muscle group, accustomed to repeated contraction throughout the day. To make them grow, you have to fatigue them much more than they're used to.'

33

IT'S ALL IN THE HIPS

How does proper hip rotation increase your ability to most effectively target the lower abs?

'The movement required to contract the lower abs is very small, and a common mistake is to continue the movement beyond its useful limits.'

A: Abdominal training — especially that of the lower region — is one of the least understood yet most talked-about training topics. Well-developed upper abs get you noticed, but equal attention to the bottom half is required for any serious bodybuilder or other athlete. An understanding of how these muscles function and some tips on lower ab training will give you the necessary tools to build the midsection of your dreams.

Several muscles comprise the abdominal wall, with the rectus abdominis being the largest and most visible. This solid sheet of muscle covers the front of the torso from the sternum to the pelvis (lower hip region), and contraction of the rectus abdominis draws the hips and ribs together. Due to the muscle's length, separate training of the upper and lower regions is required for maximal development.

The movement or range of motion (ROM) required to contract the lower abs is very small, and a common mistake is to continue the movement beyond its useful limits. Avoid this — it reduces the effectiveness of the exercise and shifts the emphasis from the lower abs to the hip flexors. Certain lower abdominal exercises may be finished with extra leg movement and exaggerated hip flexion (such as the hanging leg raise), but most should be restricted to pelvic rotation.

To target the lower abs, keep your upper body stationary and curl your hips toward your ribs, as in a reverse crunch or hanging leg raise. Think of your hips as

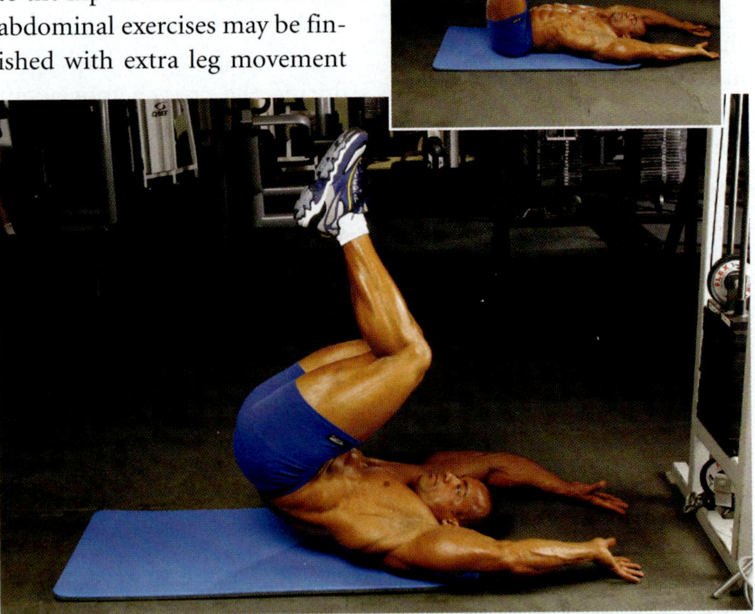

When doing a reverse crunch, movement comes from the hips, not the legs.

being on a swivel with a pivot point running right through the middle. When training lower abs, rotate your pelvis back (the top of the pelvis moves back while the bottom moves forward) as if you were trying to tuck your butt in or flatten your lower back. Hip flexion is inherent to any lower ab exercise, but concentrating on movement from the hips, not the legs, minimizes the involvement. Remember, the ROM necessary to target the lower abs is quite small. Focus on the intensity of the contraction rather than on moving your legs.

Abdominal exercises must be performed in a slow and controlled manner, just like most other exercises. A controlled action permits greater focus, allowing you to concentrate on 1) performing the correct movement, 2) obtaining maximal contraction, and 3) experiencing the overall "feel" of the exercise. These concepts are often neglected by novice bodybuilders but are essential for optimal isolation and development of the abdominals.

Proper breathing can further enhance the effects of good exercise mechanics. Contrary to popular belief, holding your breath and exhaling at peak contraction is more beneficial than exhaling during exertion. The held air increases intra-abdominal pressure, providing better spinal stability and improved muscle contraction. Adjusting to this breathing method will take some time, but you'll immediately feel the superior contraction you derive from the added pressure.

34

REPS & AB TRAINING

As my abdominal training has progressed, the number of repetitions necessary to fatigue my abs has increased. Should I continue increasing the number of reps, or should I do fewer reps with added resistance to build and strengthen my midsection? Currently, I'm doing about 50 reps of crunches.

A: When it comes to ab training, don't forgo common sense and basic training techniques for inappropriate methods of muscle development. The abdominal muscles are no different than other skeletal muscles, so the same principles you use to build muscle elsewhere should be used to develop a strong midsection. This goes for rep ranges as well as frequency of your workouts, too.

Along with the muscles of the lower back, the abdominals serve as postural muscles for standing and moving. They contract frequently and must remain contracted for extended periods, suggesting that they're designed for endurance activities. Research has confirmed this, showing that the abdominal muscles are generally composed of a greater percentage of endurance fibers than power fibers.[1] This "endurance" factor warrants abdominal training that incorporates a higher number of repetitions. Fifteen or even 20 reps of a given ab exercise is acceptable, but if you can do more than that, it's time to add resistance.

If you simply desire a firm, toned midsection, you don't need to limit the number of reps. If you're seeking strength

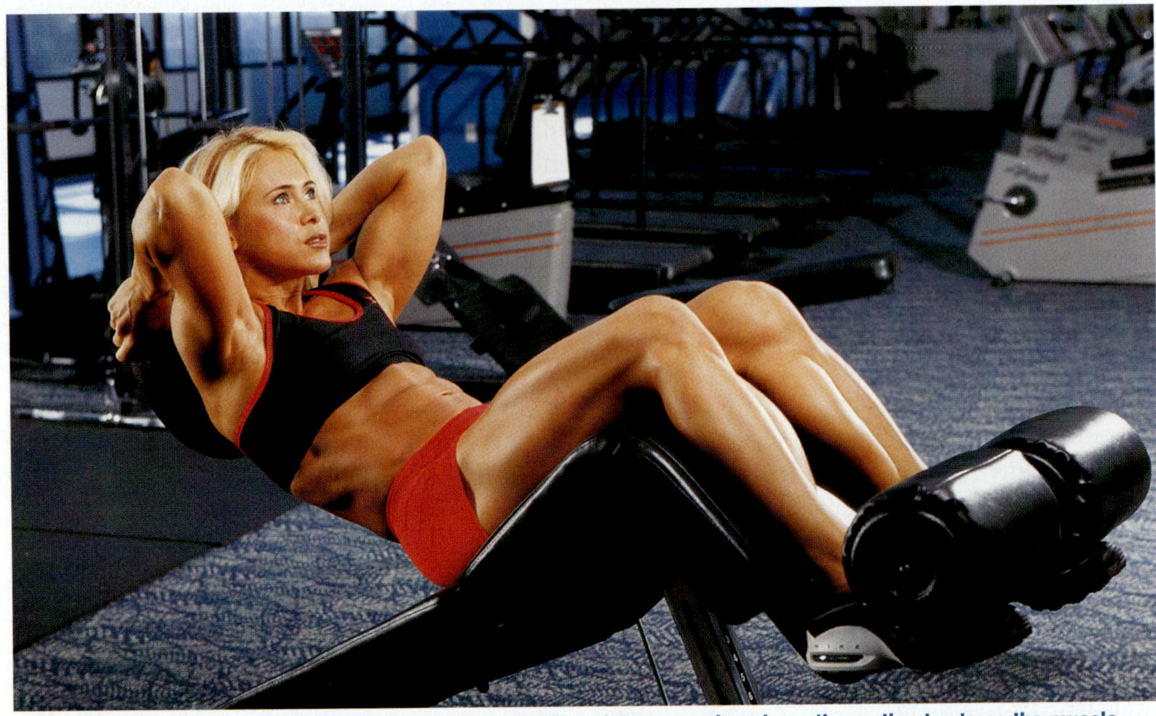

If it's easy to do 20 reps of an ab exercise, it's time to add resistance or slow down the motion to stress the muscle.

and mass, however, resistance must be continually increased to force the muscle to fatigue within a finite number of reps. Take the biceps curl as an example: You could do sets of 50 reps with a light weight, resulting in toned biceps with good endurance properties, but the muscles wouldn't be very strong and would gain very little size. The same is true for the abdominals.

To develop strength and mass, an appropriate resistance must be used to adequately stress the muscle and stimulate growth.

Yet you can increase the stress on the muscle without adding resistance. One way is to slow the motion, pausing at the end of the movement to maximally hold the contraction. Maintaining constant tension in the muscle by not resting at the top or bottom and using a controlled pace throughout the range of motion can have a similar effect. Both techniques, alone or together, will increase the intensity without increasing resistance. But to really build mass, you'll likely have to add resistance to your ab training eventually.

Care must be taken when training abs — the obliques in particular — to avoid excessive

'The abdominal muscles are no different than other muscles, so the same principles you use to build muscle elsewhere should be used to develop a strong midsection.'

mass and overdevelopment. A toned and muscled midsection is the focal point of a shapely and symmetrical physique. On the other hand, a massive and bulky abdomen makes the waist look wider, erasing the "V" taper and creating the illusion of narrow shoulders. Once you've laid a decent foundation of hard abdominal muscle, consider switching to a maintenance routine by reducing the frequency and intensity of your ab training. This is what many top bodybuilders do, which is why they can get by with little or no ab work at all.

Whatever you do, don't throw basic bodybuilding principles out the window just because you're training abs. The same techniques that build massive bi's and thighs will lead to the development of a strong, rippled midsection.

(35)

ISOLATING ABS

A: Body mechanics actually make it impossible to isolate any given muscle group, including the abdominal muscles. While you must accept the fact that ab training will always incorporate the hip flexors to a certain degree, you should realize that hip-flexor involvement can be minimized. If you understand the actions of the abdominal and hip-flexor muscles, you'll be able to increase the effectiveness of your ab training while limiting hip-flexor use.

The abdominal wall consists of several muscles. The one most visible when bodyfat is low, the rectus abdominis forms the cov-

eted "six-pack" down the front of the midsection. Although part of one long muscle, the upper and lower sections of the rectus abdominis are typically trained independently, as if they were separate muscles. Remember, however, that you can't completely isolate one region from another.

A common misconception about the rectus abdominis is that contraction causes flexion at the waist, as in forward bending. In fact, the rectus abdominis doesn't cross beneath the pelvis and therefore serves to compress the abdomen through spinal flexion or forward curling of the lower spine. The most effective tool in abdominal training is to visualize your abs shortening as you bring your pelvis and ribcage together.

Flexion at the waist, on the other hand, is controlled by a group of muscles collectively known as the hip flexors. The psoas major is the primary hip flexor, but the psoas minor and

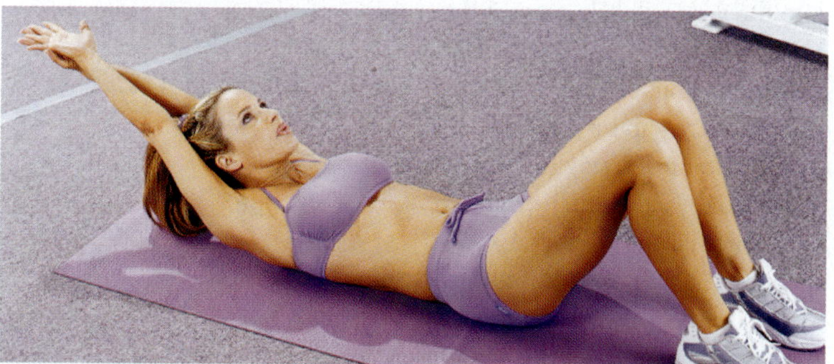

To prevent hip flexor and lower back involvement, press your lower back to the mat.

'To reduce hip-flexor involvement and lessen its pull on your lower back, bend your knees slightly.'

iliacus are also involved, to a lesser degree. Training the hip flexors is important for athletes, but excessive involvement during abdominal training detracts from the purpose of the exercise and can even lead to injury.

The psoas muscles attach to the femur (top of the thigh) and lower lumbar region (lower back). As you lie on your back with your legs straight, the psoas muscles extend, pulling on the vertebrae of the lower back. Performing abdominal movements from this position puts undue stress on your lower back and greatly increases the risk of injury by means of hyperextension, or excessive arching. To reduce hip-flexor involvement and lessen its pull on your lower back, bend your knees slightly. Additionally, flattening your lower back by pressing it into the floor will help prevent the hip flexors from arching the lower back. Although effective, this movement requires a great deal of lower abdominal strength.

Effective abdominal training with minimal hip-flexor involvement can be summarized this way:

• Whether you're training upper or lower abs, first bring your knees slightly toward your chest to lessen hip-flexor involvement and reduce pull on your lower back.

• Flatten your lower back and hold that position throughout the exercise to prevent the hip flexors from pulling the spine out of place.

• For upper-ab movements, think about bringing your ribcage toward your pelvis by maximally shortening the rectus abdominis. For lower-ab exercises, think about bringing your pelvis toward your ribcage by doing the same.

36

Lat Training Simplified

Normally I do pull-downs for my lats, but I've heard from a few sources that you need to train this muscle with several different movements to achieve complete development. It's my understanding that, unlike quads or delts, the lats have only one head. Why, then, do I need to train different parts of the muscle with different actions?

A: True, the latissimus dorsi is not composed of several heads like other significant muscles (deltoids, quadriceps, triceps, biceps). However, it is a sizable triangle-shaped muscle spanning each side of your lower and middle back with extensive and complex origins. As you'll soon see, anatomy and muscle mechanics dictate that using a selection of exercises to maximally stress this muscle group from a variety of directions is crucial for complete development. In addition, using various exercises in your routine ensures you'll hit all the muscles of your back, including the teres major and minor, infraspinatus, rhomboids and the erector spinae.

Each lat originates along the hip and lower spine, and gradually narrows until its insertion point near the end of the humerus (the upper arm bone) closest to your shoulder joint. Due to the expansive origin of this muscle, the fibers run in different directions; the upper fibers run almost horizontally, the middle fibers tend to be angled upward and the lower fibers run vertically upward. So, although it is a single muscle mass, dividing the lat into upper and lower regions based on this fiber distribution simplifies the training process by making it easier to associate exercises with each region.

The upper portion of the lat is the "wing" that fills the gap between the waist and shoulder, completing the V-taper appearance. The lower segment runs down the side and across the middle back, providing the "meat" of the lower back. Good lats drastically increase back width and girth, which are both essential for bodybuilders at any level.

Shifting Emphasis

The primary movements controlled by the lats include shoulder extension (backward movement of the arm in a vertical plane), shoulder adduction (downward movement of the arm, toward the body, in a lateral plane), medial rotation of the arm at the shoulder (turning the arm inward), and depression of the humerus (downward movement of the upper arm and shoulder).

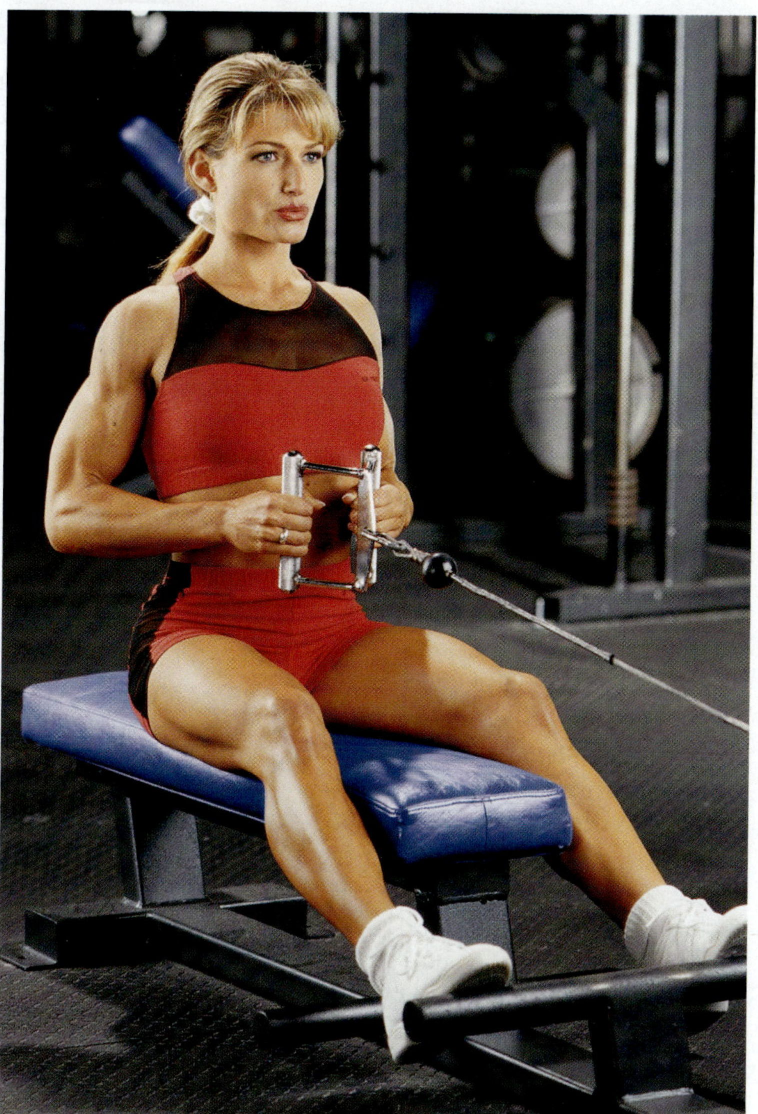

Seated rows are a great move to increase the thickness of your lower lats.

Shoulder extension works the lower lats most directly; shoulder adduction predominantly hits the upper lats. If

'Good lats drastically increase back width and girth, which are both essential for bodybuilders at any level.'

you can't remember which movements work which lat region, think of elbow position. Exercises for upper lats begin with the elbows up and out to your sides. The starting position for lower-lat exercises is with elbows in front of the body, shoulder-width apart. Regardless of which area you're targeting, finish each lat movement by pulling your elbows down and back to depress the shoulder blades.

Popular exercises for the upper lats include pull-ups and pull-downs with a wide and/or pronated (palms facing outward) grip. These same exercises can be modified to stress the lower lats by assuming a narrow, neutral (palms facing each other) or supinated (palms toward face) grip. Additionally, the pull-down's emphasis is shifted from upper to lower lat as you lean backward and pull farther down the torso, such as to the abdomen instead of the upper chest.

Rowing movements, whether seated or bent-over barbell/ dumbbell exercises, are the bread and butter of lower-lat growth. Hand placement and grip width change the emphasis of the row slightly, but not to the extent that they do with the pull-down. The pull-over is another good exercise for lower-lat development.

As you can see, a handful of basic lat exercises can be turned into a virtually unlimit-

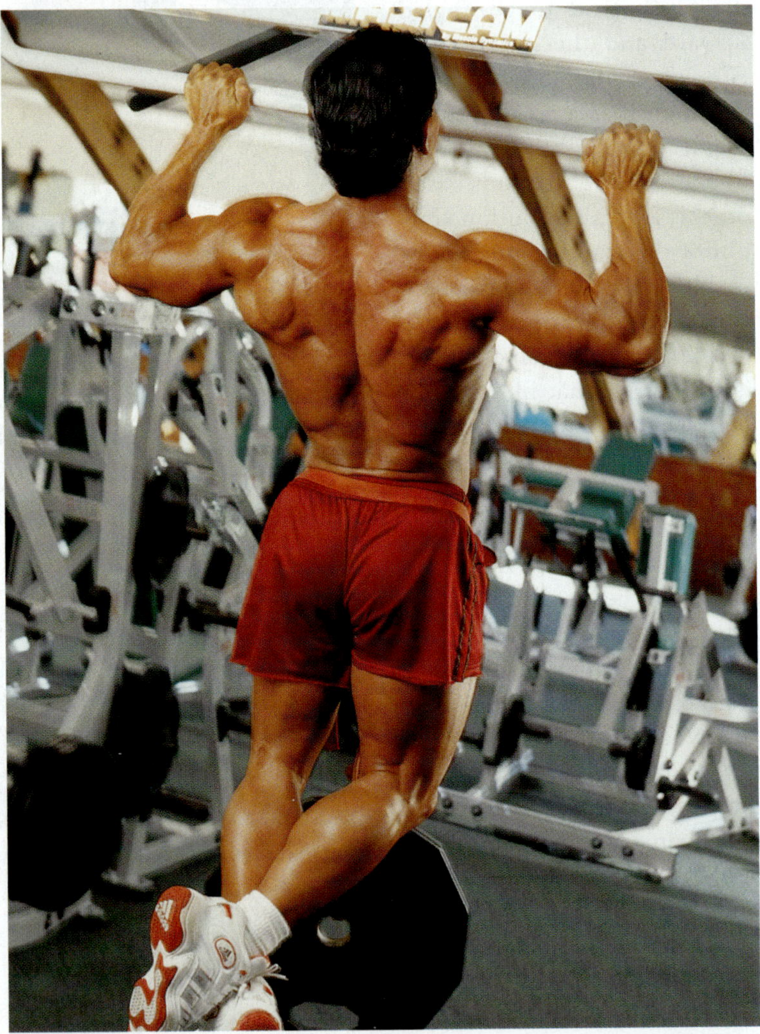

Performing pull-ups with a wide and overhand grip stresses the upper lats.

ed number of movements with simple modifications to hand position and grip width. Such changes might seem trivial, yet each change, no matter how small, stresses the muscle differently. This, in turn, emphasizes different areas, incorporates different muscle fibers and ultimately leads to more complete development.

PULL-UPS VS. CHIN-UPS

I've read that using your bodyweight as resistance is a great way to build your back. Which bodyweight exercise — chin-ups or pull-ups — is better for developing the muscles in my back?

A: The terms "chin-up" and "pull-up" are often used interchangeably, even though they are two distinctly different exercises. The muscles worked are essentially

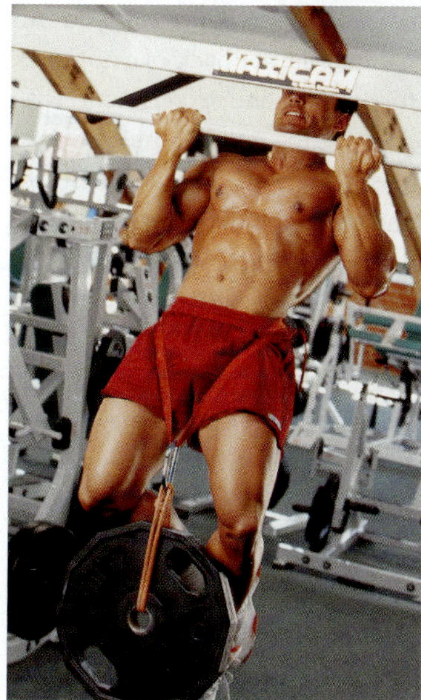

Chin-ups hit the lower lats hard.

the same for each, but the emphasis is significantly different for certain key muscles.

The distinguishing and most visible difference between the chin-up and pull-up is hand position: The chin-up uses a supinated grip (palms facing your body) whereas the pull-up uses a pronated grip (palms facing away). Standard grip width for the chin-up is shoulder-width or less, while a shoulder-width or wider grip is customary for pull-ups.

Except for the trapezius (traps), the muscles involved in the chin-up and pull-up are the same. The latissimus dorsi (lat) is the primary muscle group, but the pectoralis major (pecs), teres major, rhomboids and biceps are also called upon. Muscle recruitment is similar for each exercise, although the angles of stress are slightly different. Lat involvement is the notable exception, in which emphasis switches between upper and lower regions.

The supinated grip of the chin-up keeps the elbows in, making shoulder extension (movement of the upper arm down toward the body in a horizontal plane) the primary movement. Shoulder extension incorporates the lower lats, the muscled area on the sides of the middle-lower back. Near the end of the movement, as your chin approaches the bar, the rhomboids help rotate the scapulae (shoulder blades) while the middle traps adduct them (pull them together). For maximum rhomboid and traps contraction — and upper-middle

'Except for the trapezius (traps), the muscles involved in the chin-up and pull-up are the same.'

91

back development — concentrate on pulling your elbows down and back as you squeeze your shoulder blades together.

Shoulder adduction (downward movement of the upper arm toward the body in a lateral plane) is the primary movement of the pull-up due to the wide elbow position required for the pronated grip. Unlike the chin-up, there is little traps involvement with the pull-up, and emphasis is shifted to the upper lats. Upper lat development fills the gap between the waist and shoulders, giving the body great width from both the front and back while creating the much-desired V-taper. Like the chin-up, the pull-up incorporates the rhomboids at the end of the movement when the elbows are pulled down and back.

Don't worry if you can't decide whether to do chin-ups or pull-ups — you need to do both. Use chin-ups to hit the lower lats, adding thickness and meat to the sides of your middle-lower back. Chin-ups can also be useful when you want to work the biceps a little differently, even though your main concentration should be on back development.

You need to do pull-ups, too. They build the highly visible "wings" which, when developed properly, will truly separate you from other bodybuilders. To really emphasize the upper lats, you can try pulling the back of your neck to the bar and experiment with grip width. As your pull-up grip gets wider, lat tension increases and the emphasis shifts even more to the upper lat region. Range of motion consequently decreases, though, so there's a limit to how wide you can go. You'll have to experiment to find the grip width that works best for you.

38

KNOW THE ROW

Recently, I've seen a lot of people performing cable rows with little or no forward lean and upper-body movement. In the past, many hardcore bodybuilders advocated using upper-body movement to fully "stretch" the back muscles and increase the range of motion. What's the correct form and body position?

A: On the row, the goal is inner and outer development of the middle back. Adherence to strict form is a given for any exercise, yet it must be particularly stressed for rowing movements. Injury is always a concern, but incorrect execution can also limit growth, especially since so few movements work the innermost areas of the middle back.

Good form starts with proper body position. The areas of interest for rowing are the waist/lower back, shoulders and scapula (shoulder blades). The seated row will be explained here, but upper-body position is essentially the same for bent-over rows with dumbbells, barbells or a T-bar.

The row is not a lower-back

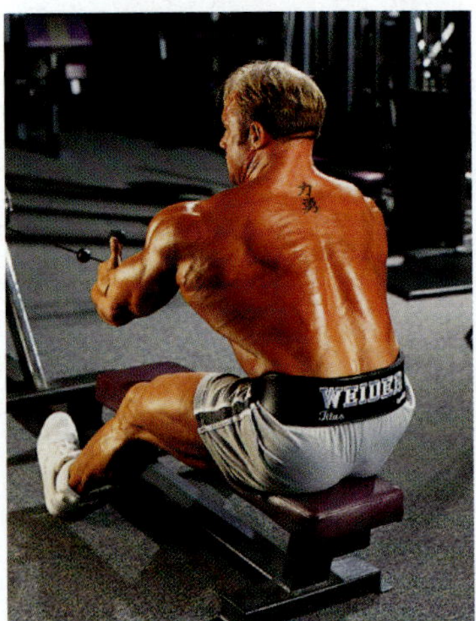

When doing a row, try not to lean forward when returning the weight.

'The seated cable row is designed to work the inner and outer portions of the middle back. It's not intended as a lower-back exercise.'

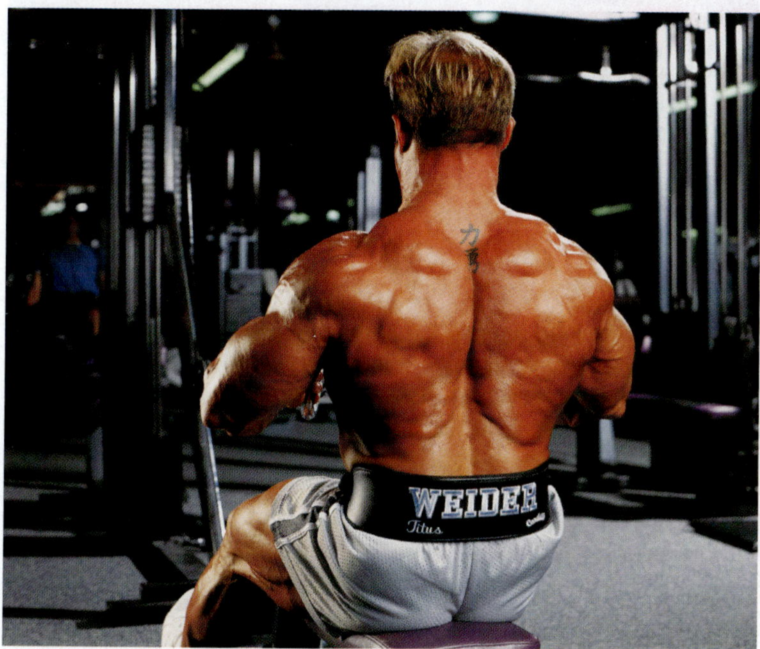

At the end position of a cable row, the shoulder blades are drawn together.

exercise. That means there should be no movement at the waist. You should not lean forward when returning the weight, nor should you lean backward as you pull the weight toward your body. Your lower back should remain stationary throughout the entire exercise. Bending at the waist decreases the effectiveness of the exercise by shifting the stress from the desired muscles (middle back) to the lower back. It also increases the risk of lower-back injury.

The shoulders and shoulder blades, on the other hand, should experience movement during the row. In the start position — with arms outstretched in front of you — the shoulders should be rolled forward and the shoulder blades spread wide. The latissimus dorsi (lats) are the primary muscles involved as you begin to pull back. As your arms pass your sides and move behind your body, the middle trapezius (traps) pulls the shoulder blades together while the rhomboideus major and minor (rhomboids) rotate them downward. At the finish of the movement, your elbows should be down and back, causing your shoulders and shoulder blades to come together as close as possible.

On the other hand, if you keep your shoulder blades completely retracted during the return of the weight to the start position, the traps are essentially removed from the exercise and rhomboid involvement is severely limited. True, both muscle groups remain in a state of isometric contraction, but range of motion is decreased to nearly nothing while muscle fiber recruitment is significantly reduced. Make sure you allow your shoulders to round forward to maximize both trap and rhomboid involvement and development. However, resist the temptation to bend at the waist or round your low back as your shoulders roll forward.

Grip has a minor effect on muscle involvement and virtually

no effect on exercise mechanics. The neutral grip (palms facing each other) permits the elbows to stay close to your sides and requires greater trap recruitment. A pronated grip (palms facing the floor) forces the elbows out, causing more direct involvement from the posterior deltoid (rear shoulder). Both grips should be used to introduce variety and stress the muscles from slightly different angles.

KEEP 'EM SEPARATED

Every time I train back, my biceps wear out before I feel anything in my lats. While this is great for my biceps, my lats are lagging. Can any exercise maximize stress on the lats with minimal involvement of the biceps?

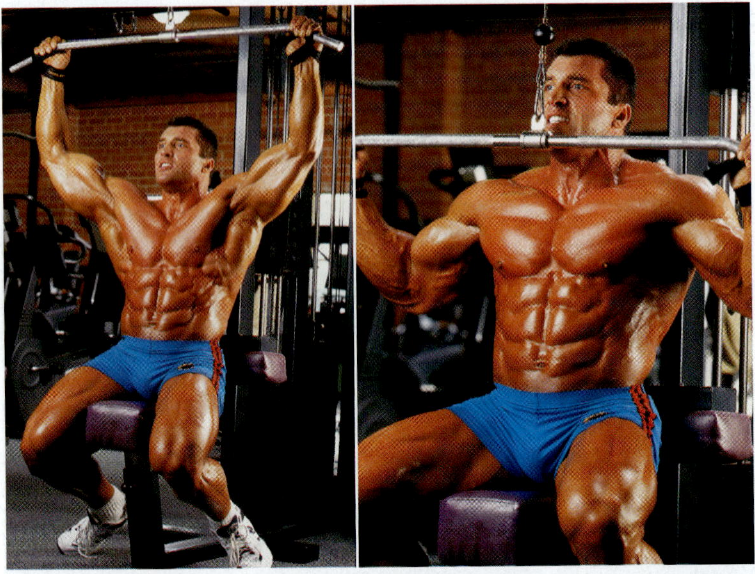

A wide grip decreases the involvement of your biceps during a pull-down.

A: As so often is the case, the answer to your question is based on anatomy and biomechanics. Probably one of the most important points you should understand is that your body works as a unit, meaning that you can't do any exercise and expect it to work only one muscle. If we're talking about a multijoint movement, such as most lat exercises, the number of muscles that come into play is even greater.

Lat movements typically require you to bring your arms from an above-the-head position down to your sides, as in any pull-down or pull-up; or in the case of rowing motions, to bring your arms from a position in front of your body to behind your body. The key is that one of your lats' primary functions is to bring your arms from an extended position down to your body. But guess what? Your pecs do so as well, and since you have to bend your arms at the elbows, all your elbow flexors (biceps, brachialis and brachioradialis) are involved, too. This is where your body really works as a unit and why you feel your biceps working hard when you train lats.

Another crucial concept in the "body as a unit" equation is that irrespective of what you might feel, all of these muscles are working. In other words, you simply can't do a pull-up or row without contracting your arm flexors. Well, at least you wouldn't get a full range of motion out of it. The flip side to this is that even though you seem to feel your biceps more, your lats are still contributing a great deal to the exercise; if they didn't, you wouldn't be able to complete it.

Now, you might be asking yourself: "That's fine, but if my biceps are so involved and they aren't strong enough to 'hang,' don't I have a problem?" Here's your favorite answer: It depends on how you look at it. Maybe you can't take your lats to the limit because your bi's aren't strong enough. On the other hand, since your bi's aren't strong enough to complete a tough set, your lats must be working harder.

pull-ups require you to bend your elbows more to get a full range of motion, which involves your biceps greatly. Using a wide grip decreases the range of motion around your elbow and therefore decreases biceps involvement. This also increases the degree to which your upper arms come down to your sides, which equals greater lat involvement.

Another function of your lats is to bring your arms from an above-the-head position to straight down in front of you and below your waist. You can mimic this movement in the straight-arm pull-down. Consider using a rope instead

'Your body works as a unit, meaning that you can't do any exercise and expect it to work only one muscle.'

The answer to your dilemma lies in program design and a little more anatomy. For one, train your bi's as hard as any muscle group. The stronger they get, the bigger and more conditioned they'll be, though you might want to give yourself a few days of rest before you train back. Also consider that close-grip pull-downs and

of a straight bar in an attempt to bring your arms past your body for greater lat work.

In the final analysis, just because you feel your bi's more than your lats doesn't mean your lats aren't working. At the same time, if you make some minor alterations in your training, you might be able to emphasize your lats more.

40

TARGETING BI'S

How can I make my biceps rounded on the top? They seem to be getting larger, but what's the best exercise to achieve a ball effect?

A: If you look at an anatomy chart, you'll notice that the biceps has two fairly distinct heads. The reason lies in the fact that this muscle originates from two different areas on your shoulder blade — the coracoid process for the short head and the supraglenoid tubercle for the long head — yet it inserts with a common tendon on your forearm (on the radius bone). If you don't have an anatomy chart, just check out a picture of Ronnie Coleman. You can easily see the two heads; the short head's on the inside, the long head's on the outside.

The ball effect you're talking about is due to superior long head development. The obvious question is, how do you attain that? Let's delve a bit deeper into anatomy and science to find an answer.

'Stick to basic, heavy barbell and dumbbell curls to get as much overall growth as you possibly can.'

Anatomically and biomechanically, the biceps flexes the elbow, supinates the forearm (twisting your wrist so that your palm faces up), stabilizes the front of the shoulder and flexes the shoulder (albeit weakly). With this in mind, researchers from the department of biomedical science at the University of Wollongon, Australia, tried to

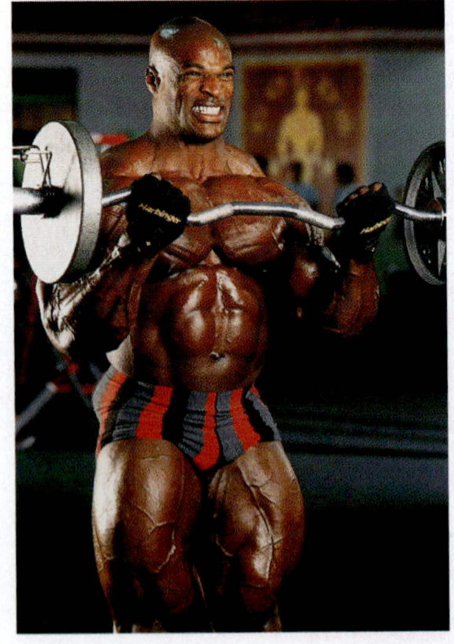

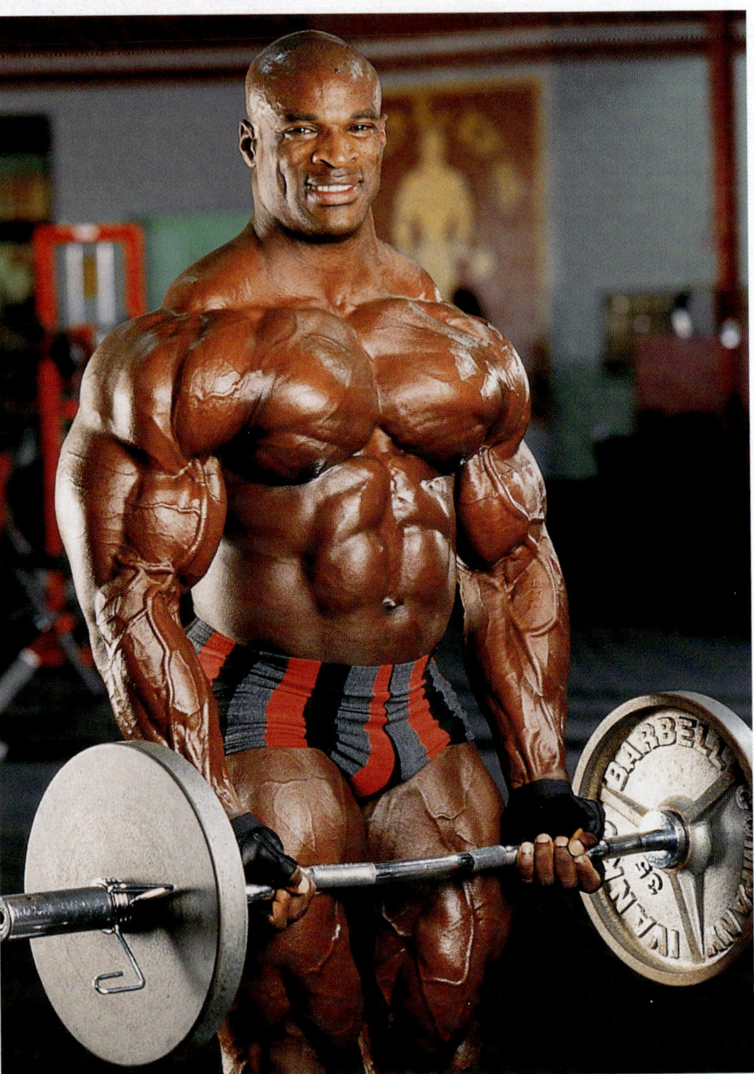

Though genetics plays a key role, you'll see a greater peak from superior long head development. Heavy barbell curls will get you that growth.

determine if the two heads of the biceps could be separately activated during supination at different levels of elbow bend. They found that the degree of elbow bend had more effect on differential contractions than the amount of weight lifted. They also learned that if you completely bend your elbow and supinate your wrist, the short head is more active. Conversely, as the angle of elbow bend decreases, the long head becomes more involved.

This drives home the point of emphasis over isolation. Both parts of the biceps were active, but one slightly more than the other depending on the movement. Again, we're left to wonder if that would translate into noticeably more size in one part over the other. Hard to say, but we'll still give it a shot.

So, how should you train? Stick to basic, heavy barbell and dumbbell curls — either standing, seated or on a preacher bench — to get as much overall growth as you possibly can. At the end of the workout, consider holding a fairly heavy dumbbell and rotating your wrist while keeping a 30–40-degree angle in your elbow.

41

TWIST OF THE WRIST

I see people at the gym rotating their hands when they do dumbbell curls for biceps and flyes for chest. Is this just a matter of preference or does some muscular benefit exist?

A: Whereas for some bodybuilders it might be a matter of preference, turning your wrist does in fact slightly change the angle of stress placed upon the muscle and, in some cases, modifies the degree of muscle involvement. This technique can be incorporated into curling, pressing (shoulder or chest) and flye movements using dumbbells or cables. The most direct benefits are derived during biceps curls; effects are less significant for overhead presses, and decrease further for flyes.

When you stand with your hands at your sides, palms facing each other, your hands are in what's called a neutral position. Turning your hand and forearm out so your palm is facing forward is called supination. The opposite motion — with

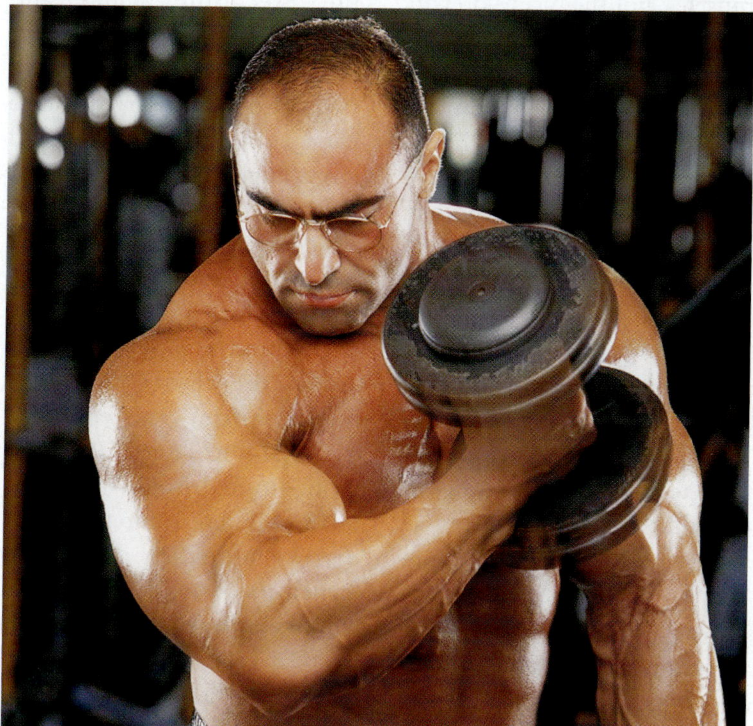

Twisting the wrist during curls results in a more complete biceps contraction.

'By supinating your hand during the upward phase of the biceps curl, you perform both flexion and supination.'

your hand and forearm turned in until your palm faces backward — is called pronation.

The standard biceps curl targets the biceps brachii, brachialis and brachioradialis muscles, but the biceps brachii and brachioradialis also supinate the lower arm. By supinating your hand during the upward phase of the biceps curl, you simultaneously perform both flexion and supination. The result is a more complete contraction of the flexors and involvement of the supinator muscle. Turning your hand inward as you lower it to the starting position incorporates the pronator muscles while continuing to work the brachioradialis.

Adding this simple twisting motion to a standard biceps curl can lead to increased mass in the biceps muscle and enhanced development of the brachioradialis and pronator teres muscles. The pronator teres is located at the upper-inside portion of the forearm; the brachioradialis is highly visible on the upper-outside of the forearm. Development of both results in forearms worthy of the nickname Popeye.

Pronation or supination can also be used in the overhead press, bench press or flye, but the resistance against the forearm muscles is reduced due to the execution angles and forces of gravity. For these movements, pronation and supination primarily cause changes in elbow position and stress angle.

Supination during the overhead press brings the elbows in, moving the stress toward the anterior (front) portion of the deltoid muscle. Pronation makes the elbows flare outward, shifting the emphasis back to the lateral (middle) head of the deltoid.

In a similar fashion, supination or pronation during the bench press or flye moves the elbows inward or outward, respectively. Elbow position doesn't dramatically affect muscle involvement, but will alter the angle of pull and contraction. Executing these movements with various hand positions ensures the greatest degree of muscle involvement and overall development, but make sure you get the hang of such twists with relatively light weights before going heavy.

42

BENCH-PRESS DIFFERENCES

If you use the same amount of weight, would you see any difference in results between using a machine or barbell for bench pressing? I don't have a spotter, so I usually just use the machines, but I heard that you can't gain mass unless you use a barbell. Is this true?

A: For the most part, machines shouldn't severely limit your development. Yet if you're an elite athlete or advanced bodybuilder and want to maximize your development, free weights may deliver better. But first, we commend you on doing the smart thing when a spotter isn't available. Whatever development differences may occur by using a machine vs. a barbell, it won't really mean a whole heck of a lot if you end up with a barbell across your neck, literally turning you into a pencilneck.

You might be limiting your gains, however, by using the same weight in each movement. The amount of weight you can lift or the number of reps you can perform usually depends on the type of apparatus you use. Different mechanics and even something as simple as grip-width changes can make a difference.[2,3]

Some research also indicates that relatively inexperienced male subjects' max lifts were more with free weights than with a Universal machine, though the difference wasn't significant.[4] Alternatively, research presented at the 1998 National Strength & Conditioning Association's Annual Conference found that using a Hammer Strength isolateral chest press produced almost equal changes in max strength and fat-free mass over a 10-week training period as a free-weight bench press in fairly inexperienced subjects.[5] In other words, machine designs vary, and you can't expect equal results from machine to machine.

Basically, you can't predict across the board that you'll always lift more with free weights vs. a machine, or vice versa. So you'd probably be better off changing the weight depending on the intensity or effort called for by the day's workout.

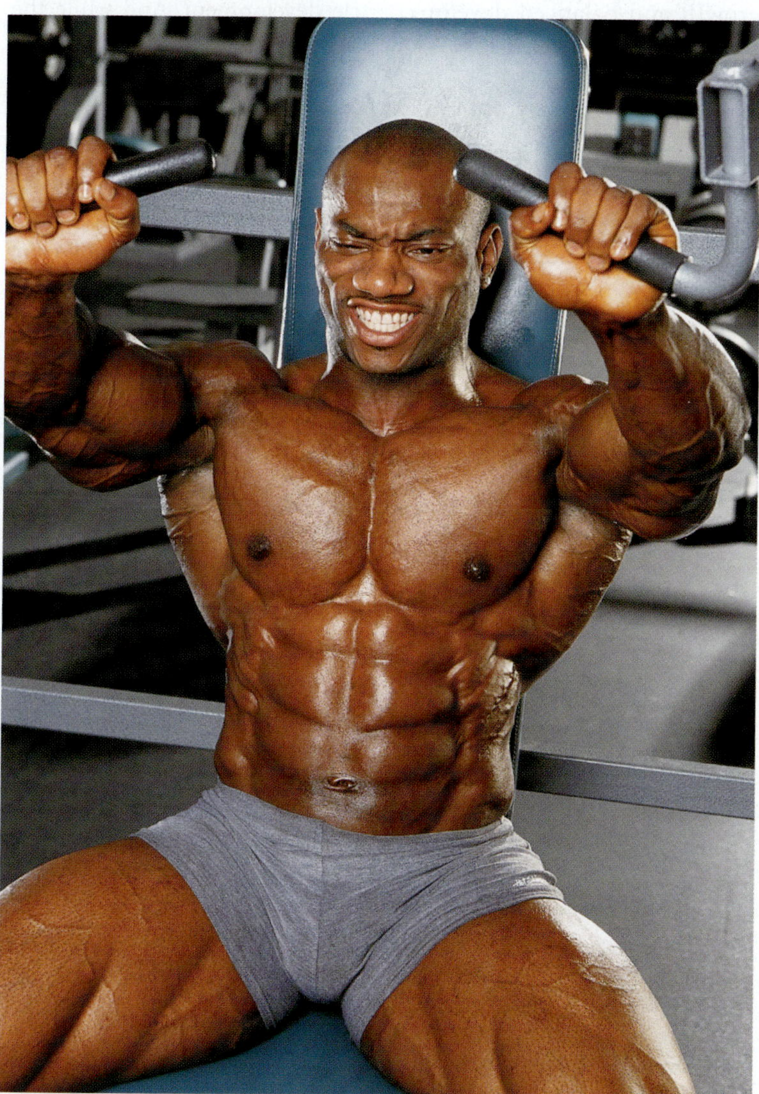
Unless you're a beginner, you may want to limit machine bench presses.

In terms of relative differences between a free-weight and machine bench press, you can't expect the exact same gains. As an example, researchers from McMaster University in Hamilton, Ontario, Canada, found that single-joint exercises produced a quicker growth response in beginners than multijoint exercises.[6] They didn't specifically look at the machine vs. free-weight bench press, but one conclusion was that your muscles can start growing sooner via easier single-joint movements than if you had to spend a lot of time learning how to do a more complex multijoint exercise. The comparison is between the relative ease of benching in a machine over using free weights. As you well know, the machine will dictate your movement, there's no learning curve and you don't have to worry about balance, coordination, etc.

So on one hand — particularly if you're a beginner or intermediate bodybuilder — it doesn't seem that machine benches will result in tremendous differences in strength and size over free-weight bench presses. If you're an advanced bodybuilder who wants to maximize your gains, however, consider limiting machine benches to those times when a spotter isn't available. Since free-weight benches are more difficult to perform, the recruitment of more muscles will result in more overall growth and balanced development for you.

43

BENCH-PRESS ROM

What is the proper technique for the bench press? How can I avoid the lingering shoulder injuries that so many lifters have acquired?

A: As with any exercise, performing the bench press properly through its full range of motion (ROM) is important for complete muscle development. And while the bench press is a relatively simple movement, you must use caution to prevent injury at the extreme ends of the exercise. A good working knowledge of bench-press mechanics and proper execution will enable you to safely get the most from the "big daddy" of chest exercises.

Muscle Involvement

The principal muscles involved in the bench press are the pectoralis major (pecs), anterior deltoids and the triceps. Several other muscles of

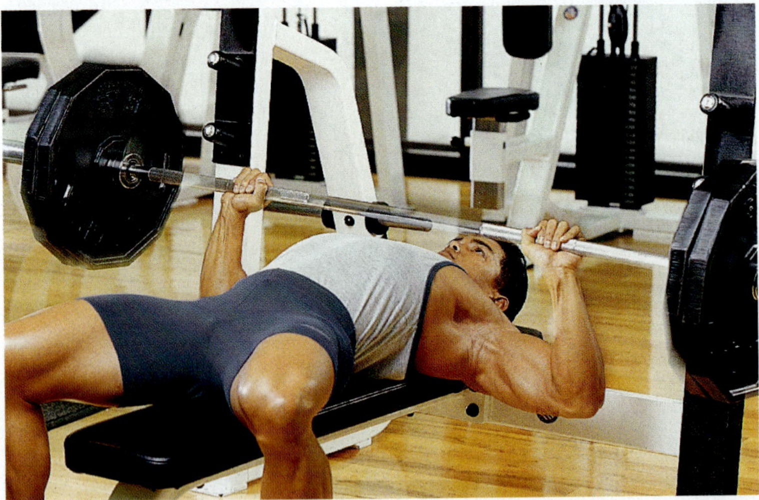

Pulling your shoulders back will stretch out your pecs and extend your ROM.

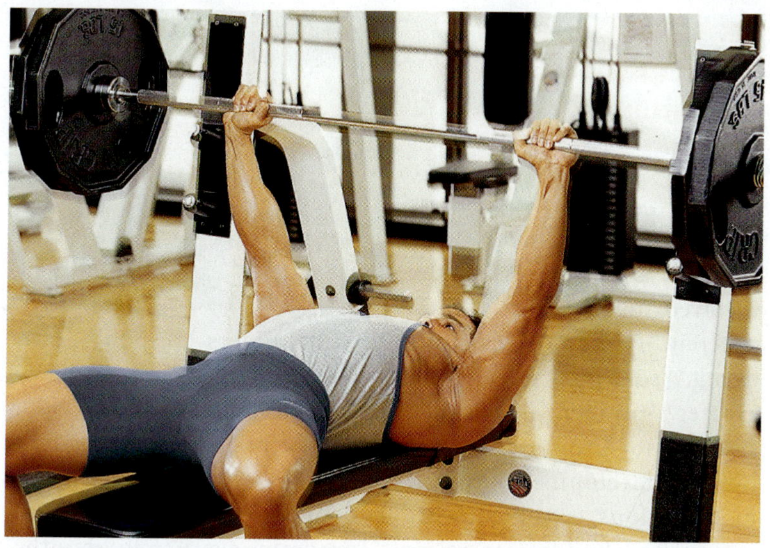

In the finish position, the bar should be over your shoulders, not your pecs.

the chest, back and shoulders are involved as assistors and/or stabilizers, but pec development is the primary goal.

Horizontal adduction — movement of the outstretched arm across and in front of the body — is the most direct movement utilizing the pectoralis major. Usually, using a barbell limits the degree of horizontal adduction but provides greater safety and allows the use of heavier weights. In most cases, horizontal adduction should not exceed the midline of the body (your elbow shouldn't pass below the level of your shoulder). Beyond this point, emphasis of the movement shifts from the pec muscles to the shoulder joints, a sit-uation that's neither beneficial nor desirable. Yet individuals who have longer arms or flatter chests who have been instruct-ed to touch their chests with the bar will often commit this biomechanical crime.

right ROM endpoint for every-one, however. Depending on your physical dimensions and the length of your limbs, touching the bar to your chest might exceed your physical limits. Most importantly, your shoulders should be pulled back (like you're trying to pinch your shoulder blades together) to put your pecs in a prestretched position and extend the ROM. This simple move is crucial for maintaining tension in the pecs throughout the movement and eliminates the need to extend the ROM by opening the shoulder joints.

Just as excessive horizontal adduction can put undue stress on the shoulders, a grip that's too wide or too narrow can do the same thing. Ideally, the prop-er grip width will put approxi-

'A barbell limits the degree of horizontal adduction but allows the use of heavier weights.'

Upper & Lower Limits

The start and finish positions of the bench press define its ROM. The downward move-ment of the press depends on chest size, as the bar can only be lowered until it meets the chest. This isn't necessarily the

mately a 90-degree angle in the elbow joints when the upper arms are in the bottom position (about parallel to the floor). If you're uncertain, play it safe by stopping the downward move-ment when your elbows pass the back of your shoulders.

After you hit the bottom of your ROM, push the bar up and back slightly so the finish position is over your shoulders (rather than over the lower portion of your pecs). If you push the bar straight up, the tension shifts from your pecs to your triceps. At the top of the movement your arms should be fully extended, but not locked, to keep tension on the muscles.

Final Word

The bench press is a safe and useful exercise for chest growth. Dumbbell and cable movements are good supplemental exercises for increased ROM and overall development. But more isn't always better, so be careful not to take any movement farther than your body can safely tolerate.

44

INCLINE & DECLINE

When doing chest press movements on adjustable benches, I see some people train at low angles and others at higher angles. How much difference does the degree of angle make in overall development?

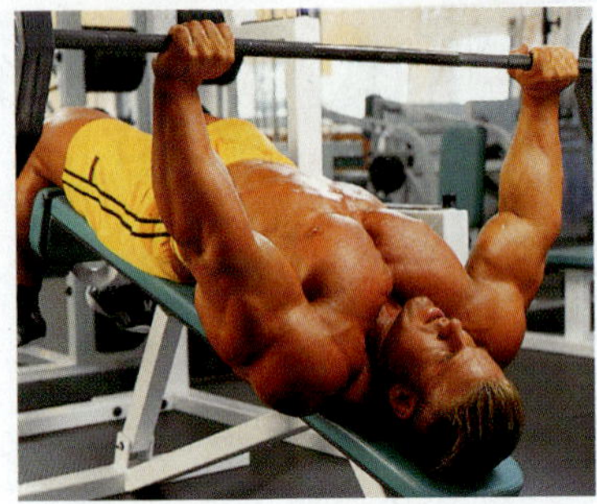

A: Changing the bench angle alters your body position, stressing the involved muscles in a slightly different fashion. Over time, doing so incorporates a greater number of muscle fibers and promotes better overall development. Minor modifications or adjustments to core bodybuilding exercises are a great way to introduce variety into your workouts without making significant changes to established, mass-building movements.

I often wonder how some bodybuilders respond after repeatedly being told to change their exercise program on a regular basis. I envision bodybuilders with good potential floundering as they start a new program every few months. Don't get me wrong — change is certainly good — but drastic modifications sometimes do more harm than good. That's where subtle changes like bench position can make a

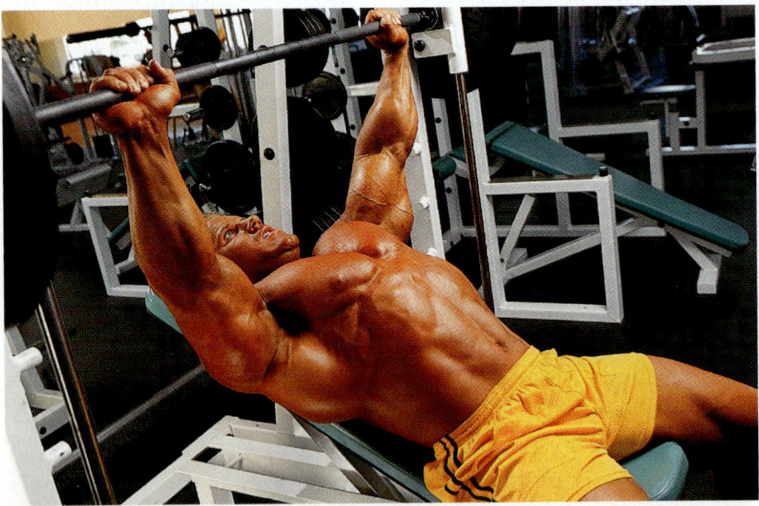

The decline bench (top of page) lets you more thoroughly work your lower pecs, while the incline bench (above) helps you hit your upper pecs and delts.

world of difference.

Let's say you've faithfully included the bench press in your workout for several months but aren't getting the fullness and definition in your chest that you desire. Instead of deleting the exercise from your program, why not modify it to target your weak areas, ultimately fulfilling your training goals?

The primary target of the bench press is the pectoralis major (pec) muscle. The standard chest press movement, performed on a flat bench, is the most direct way to work the entire pec muscle. But because the muscle is so large, attached to the chest from the clavicle all the way down to the sixth rib, it's difficult to maximally contract the entire muscle with a single movement in a single plane of motion.

A raised bench slightly shifts the emphasis of the movement from the middle portion of the pecs to the upper region; development of the upper pecs results in a chest that appears more massive. The incline position also involves the deltoid (shoulder) muscles to a greater extent and therefore serves as a good exercise for the shoulder-chest tie-in.

Performing the chest press on a decline, with the head of the bench lowered slightly (from the flat position), causes greater stimulation of the lower pec region, though there's some debate as to the degree. This is where the belly of the muscles lies, so developing this area leads to a chest that's thicker and has the appearance of greater separation from the abdomen.

When muscles are forced to contract in a way they aren't accustomed to, muscle fibers are recruited in a somewhat different manner, and incorporating more muscle fibers increases the potential for growth. Additionally, large muscle groups (chest, back, legs) must be trained from different angles to involve fibers from all parts of the muscle. Just be careful not to take the adjustable bench positions to extremes, and make sure you start out light to get the hang of movements at angles you aren't quite familiar with.

45

LOWER-PEC DILEMMA

Everything I read about chest training and kinesiology states that the lower chest is almost never underdeveloped, due to bench presses, flyes and other mass-building exercises. Unfortunately, I seem to be the exception to this rule. What can I do to bring out more size and roundness to this area? Do you think decline pressing is the answer?

A: You're right: the lower aspect of the pecs rarely lacks in development. Remember, however, that we're all built slightly different. The lower part of the chest attaches

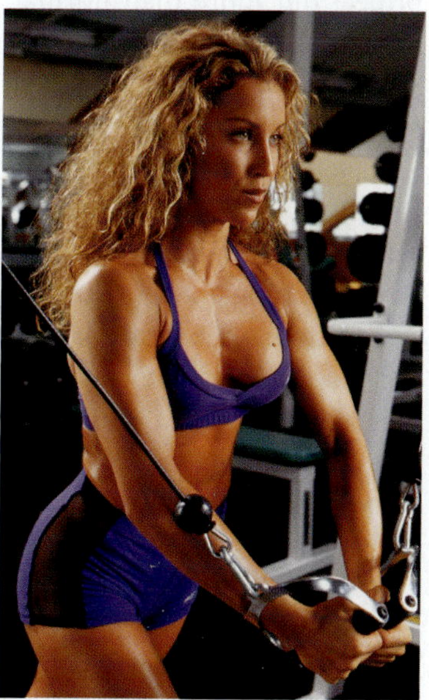

You should include cable movements for a more complete pec routine.

'For your pecs, flyes and cable movements are great choices, and try to include heavy bench presses to stimulate maximal strength development.'

to the breastbone and ribs and is called the sternocostal head of the pectoralis major. Normally your pecs attach to the upper six costal cartilages, which in turn attach the ribs to the breastbone. In your case, the lower part of your pecs may originate from the upper four or five costal cartilages, a higher-than-normal attachment that could partly explain your problem. But it might also be that your lower costal cartilages project out more than normal. Either case would translate into your lower-chest area appearing less developed.

In your attempt to shape your lower pecs, you're obviously looking for certain exercises to target that region. Yet you need to realize that the shape of your muscles is largely dictated by genetics. That is, you can't change how your muscles attach to bone and, in the case of your pecs, where the sternocostal head attaches and/or how much your costal cartilages protrude. This doesn't mean you can't get bigger and stronger, but it does mean that the way you'll look,

even if you add 40 pounds of muscle, is predetermined.

So does that mean you shouldn't do a variety of exercises? Heck no! Indeed, different angles of attack will elicit a specific sort of stress on your body to which it will adapt. In my opinion, this typically doesn't occur in a way you can notice with the naked eye, but nevertheless, the stress is different and so is the adaptation. With regard to decline presses, this basically means that if you participate in a sport that requires a similar movement, by all means do it. But if you look at this exercise from a bodybuilding perspective, you'll see that you have better choices.

The decline bench press does a very poor job of recruiting your pecs compared to the regular bench press or flye. Here's why: Your pecs are designed to bring your arms toward your body's midline (adduction), rotate your arms inward, draw in your arms from an extended position and push the arms and shoulders down. None of this occurs in the decline bench press

— the movement hardly meets any of the functional aspects of your pecs. In addition, the decline bench press offers a very limited range of motion due to how you lie on the bench, the bar hitting you at the tip of your breastbone or diaphragm area and you pressing the bar to completion over an approximate 5–10-inch distance. Not exactly ideal when compared to a regular bench or flye.

The main thing to remember and incorporate into your chest training — and all other muscle groups — is to make sure your exercises utilize the specific action the muscle is designed to do and allow for maximum-range-of-motion movements. For your pecs, flyes and cable movements are great choices, and try to include heavy bench presses to stimulate maximal strength development.

What you're basically left with is hard, heavy, smart chest training. When I say smart, I'm not only referring to proper exercise selection but also periodized training regimens in which you observe varying levels of volume (sets, reps) and intensity (weight lifted) in your workouts. Though you may never develop an incredibly massive lower-pec region, the overall appearance of your pecs can grow to become quite impressive as you continue pumping iron.

46

ON THE FLYE

I've noticed a lot of variation in the way people do dumbbell flyes at my gym. Some go really wide and low in the bottom position, and occasionally I notice someone turning his arms when he gets to the top. Can you tell me the best way to perform the flye?

A: Executing the dumbbell flye through a full but safe range of motion (ROM) is critical for maximal muscle-fiber activation. Stopping short on either end restricts muscle involve-

ment and inhibits growth. Arm position also affects muscle recruitment and varies the angle of stress. Here's how.

At the Bottom

How low should you go? While full ROM is important, continuing beyond the limits of functional motion can be detrimental, causing injury in some cases. Most movements have a natural start and stop point, such as the barbell curl. But due to the unique nature of the shoulder joint — it allows for movement of the arm in all directions — such is not the case with the dumbbell flye. In fact, it's easy to exceed the limits of safe execution, especially when you're trying to maximize ROM and get a full stretch at the bottom of

the movement.

The medically advised lower limit for the flye is the point at which your elbows are level with your shoulders (upper arms parallel to the floor). This limit can be slightly exceeded by most individuals, but each person's shoulder ROM is unique. Dropping your elbows below shoulder level permits greater outer pec involvement, but bears the consequence of excessive shoulder stress. For most bodybuilders, the benefits of going too low don't outweigh the risks.

How wide should you go? Most experts advise that you maintain a slight bend in your elbows throughout the exercise. Too much bend (going past 45 degrees) will turn the flye into a dumbbell press, an altogether

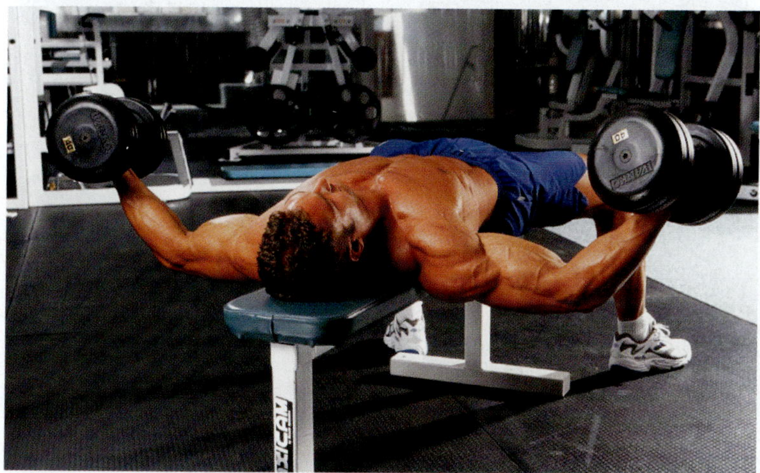

At the bottom, don't go too much lower than upper arms parallel to the floor.

different movement. On the other hand, going too wide can cause both elbow- and shoulder-joint problems. The straighter the arms, the longer the arms, and the farther you hold an object out away from your body, the greater the relative weight of that object. With completely straight arms, even the force of a 50-pound dumbbell can be excessive to the elbow and shoulder-joint complex.

At the Top

Neutral grip (palms facing each other). Most lifters complete the flye with their palms facing each other at the top. As they lower and raise the dumbbells during the exercise, their hand and arm positions remain constant. This keeps

'The advised lower limit for the flye is the point at which your elbows are level with your shoulders.'

the movement simple and effective. The added bonus is that you can generally use more weight. If you follow the theory that more weight stimulates more muscle fibers and thus leads to more growth, then this is the finish for you.

Supinated grip (palms facing your head). Some lifters swear that this method has added massive muscle to their inner pecs. While anecdotal evidence abounds, the concrete support is somewhat conflicting. To help determine if this movement is right for you, let's first

consider the biomechanics involved. By turning your arms so that your palms face toward your head, you externally rotate the humerus (upper arm bone). Because the pectoralis muscle attaches to the humerus, turning it this way lengthens the pectoralis muscle to a small degree, allowing for a slightly stronger contraction. Yet many experts will argue about the limited benefit.

Turning the arm also affects the ROM by changing the direction of the elbows. Because your elbows are slightly bent, you bring them closer together by turning your arms, thus increasing the ROM. This can be likened to the bent-arm pec-deck flye, where you concentrate on bringing your elbows together, not your hands. Much like most back exercises and lateral raises for delts, when doing flyes you need to concentrate on the movement of the elbows — not the hands. Not only can you concentrate on squeezing the pecs better, but you also reduce the involvement of the anterior deltoids.

As a final word, remember

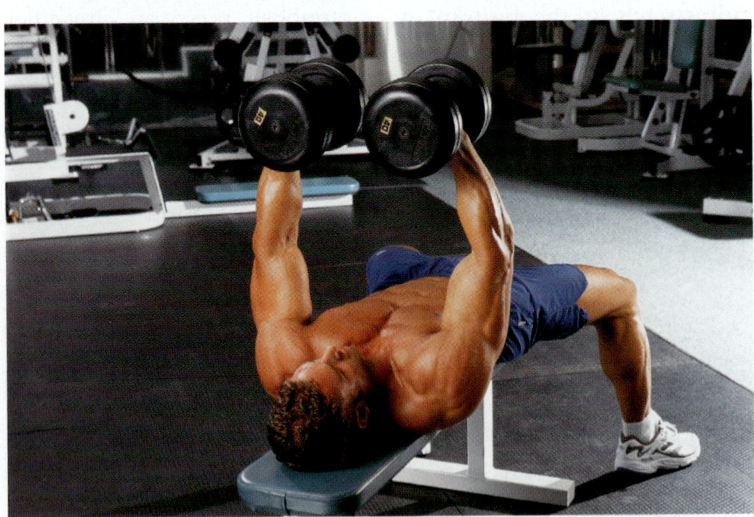

You can lift more with the neutral hand position (palms facing each other).

that neither hand position is truly better than the other. Regular use of different grips introduces variety into your chest workouts and promotes optimal pectoral growth. Just be sure to use a full but safe ROM on the dumbbell flye to keep pec development at a maximum and joint injury at a minimum.

47

PRESSING THE ISSUE

I've been doing lots of overhead and front raises, but still lack mass in my shoulders. What other exercises should I include in my shoulder workout?

A: No doubt, well-developed shoulders are the frame that encloses your masterpiece. Their thickness and width can make you look authoritative and strong, and can even create the illusion of a tiny waist.

When it comes to delt training, you really do need to shoul-

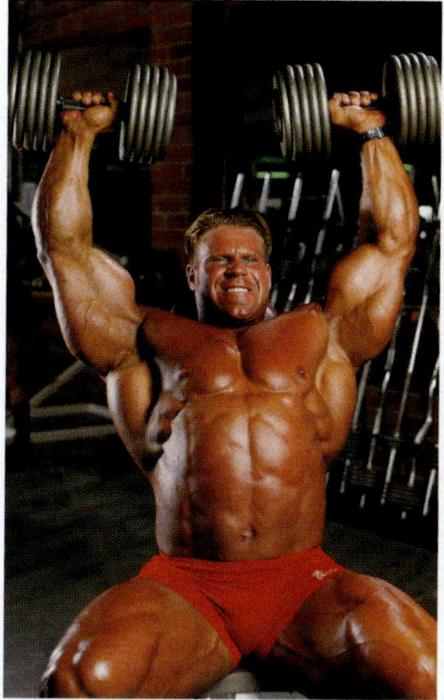

With heavy weight, seated shoulder presses are easier on your back.

der the load. In building the torso, many of us rely on chest and back exercises rather than shoulder work. That's a mistake, especially where overall symmetry and balance are concerned. The best exercises to build the delts are compound movements called presses.

Mobility vs. Stability

The shoulder press is one of the most sport-specific and functional movements in the bodybuilding repertoire. Whether you're shooting a basket or reaching for the highest shelf in your kitchen, you're using muscles involved in the shoulder press. Because this movement

is so common, it's important to properly strengthen all the muscles around the shoulder joint to avoid injury. However, this isn't as simple as just training the "show" muscles called the deltoids. The shoulder joint also contains the rotator-cuff muscles, which are relatively small, usually undertrained and quite complex.

The shoulder also works in harmony with the scapular musculature, which gives a solid base to this very mobile joint. The design of the shoulder joint allows a great degree of freedom; it has the largest range of motion of any joint in the body. Because of this mobility, though, it sacrifices some stability. By nature's design, the shoulder joint is at greater risk of injury, especially during overhead and rotational movements.

The Behind-the-Neck Controversy

An ongoing controversy over shoulder presses revolves around the potential danger of behind-neck movements with heavy loads. For some bodybuilders, using maximal weights could in fact be a problem. For most, however, following a few simple precautions will be enough to avoid

Tips on Delt Training

To get the max from your workouts and decrease your potential for injury, incorporate these tips into your delt-training program:

- Avoid training shoulders the day before or the day after chest. Your anterior deltoids will be trained two days in a row, which will result in overtraining and submaximal results.

- Training chest and shoulders together is a nice complement, but vary the bodypart trained first. If you always train chest first, your delts won't get the benefit of your full energy.

- Training back before shoulders is also a good bodypart combination because it will increase scapular stabilization and minimize injury.

- Only attempt weights you can lift with proper form. Too much weight can lead to a breakdown in form and even injury.

- With standing presses, be sure to maintain the natural curves in all areas of your back: cervical, thoracic and lumbar. If you feel yourself straining, lighten the load, switch to a seated position or do an alternate exercise.

- Seated presses are stricter and put less stress on the low back, especially with heavy weights.

- Perform unilateral and full range of motion movements for sports-specific and functional exercises.

- Monitor the number of anterior deltoid exercises performed, especially since this muscle is worked in upper-chest exercises, too.

serious injury.

Harold Reitman, MD, CSCS, CEO of Orthopaedic Associates, USA, says: "Behind-the-neck presses do put the shoulder joint in a compromised position. However, proper stretching of the chest and rotator cuff, and strengthening of the rotator cuff and scapular musculature, can reduce the chance of problems associated with this lift."

Jane Jarosz-Hlis, PT, CSCS, shoulder specialist and United States Tennis Association professional, treats athletes with shoulder injuries that stem from muscle imbalances. "The chest and anterior deltoid usually overpower the back, and this leads to poor mechanics. Then when exercises are performed incorrectly, people get hurt."

Most experts agree that any movement can be harmful if the body isn't prepared and the movement is done wrong. So before embarking on presses to expand your width, be sure to include a comprehensive stretching program that incorporates the entire upper-body musculature, especially the shoulders. In addition, do some "pre-press" training for your rotator-cuff and scapular stabilizer muscles.

48

SHOULDERING THE ROW

I'm not sure whether to include upright rows in my back or shoulder workout. Technically, would this movement be considered a deltoid or trapezius exercise?

A: Upright rows are primarily a shoulder movement, specifically meant to target the middle head of the deltoid. The trapezius is involved to a limited extent (as are the biceps), but the deltoid is the primary muscle used to properly perform the movement.

Your deltoid muscle is made up

of three heads — front, middle and rear. Each head is involved in any given shoulder movement, but specific exercises shift the emphasis slightly from one head to another. Contraction of your front deltoid raises the upper arm straight forward in a plane perpendicular to the front of your body (flexion), while contraction of your rear deltoid draws the upper arm backward (extension). When you contract your middle deltoid, your upper arm is lifted straight out to the side of your

'The key to proper execution of the upright row is hand placement and elbow movement.'

body (abduction). Well-developed middle deltoids add width to your shoulders and thus enhance the shoulder-to-waist ratio, making your waist appear more narrow.

The trapezius is a large diamond-shaped muscle that spans the width of your shoulders and runs from your neck to your lower-middle back. It is primarily responsible for movement of your scapulae (shoulder blades) in all directions. The traps also elevate your clavicle (collarbone). The upright row cannot be performed without substantial trapezius involvement, but it is secondary to deltoid contribution.

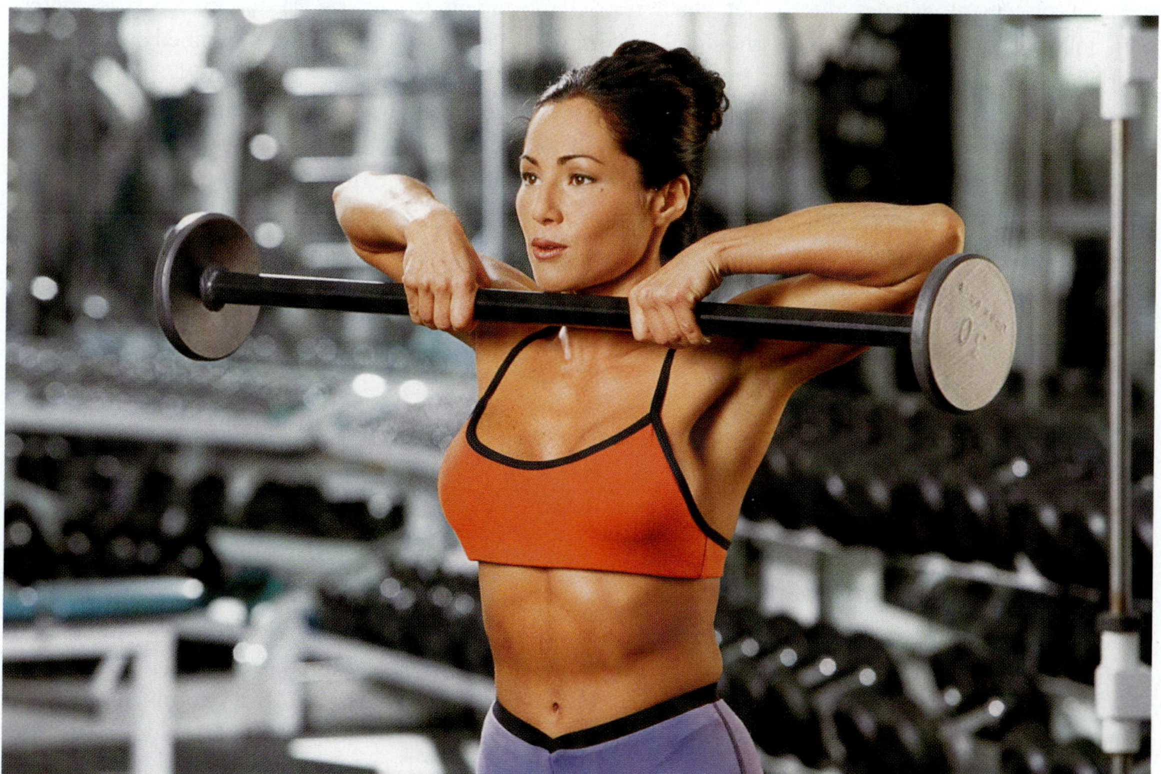

The correct hand position spreads your elbows outward, enabling you to raise them as high as possible, finishing at ear level.

The key to proper execution of the upright row is hand placement and elbow movement. Your hands should be approximately nipple-width apart — about 8 inches for most individuals — with movement initiated and led by the elbows. The middle deltoids are forced into complete contraction when the elbows are kept up, out and above the hands. Trap involvement is greatest late in the movement as the upper arms near parallel with the ground, and the shoulder blades elevate and rotate.

Hand placement dictates the path followed by the elbows. If your hands are too far apart, you'll be unable to move through a full range of motion, limiting the overall effectiveness of the exercise. A grip that's too narrow will cause your elbows to drift forward, decreasing middle deltoid involvement. The appropriate hand position spreads your elbows outward, enabling you to raise them as high as possible, nearly in line with your shoulders. Keep the bar close to your body throughout the movement to maintain a good mechanical position while decreasing the degree of stress on your lower back.

Upright rows provide a good tie-in between your shoulders and upper back, but include the exercise in your shoulder routine rather than during your back workout. You could, however, perform upright rows with back if you hit shoulders and back in the same session. Regardless, shrugs are a good follow-up exercise to hit the traps hard once they're pre-exhausted by upright rows.

To get a better "feel" for the exercise in your shoulders, try starting the movement with a shrug. By contracting the traps first, you'll then find it easier to concentrate on using the deltoids to raise your elbows. You may feel like a chicken flapping its wings, but you'll restrict movement to the shoulder joint while gaining a better understanding of the exercise. Practice this variation with lighter weights to ensure proper form and to become accustomed to the movement.

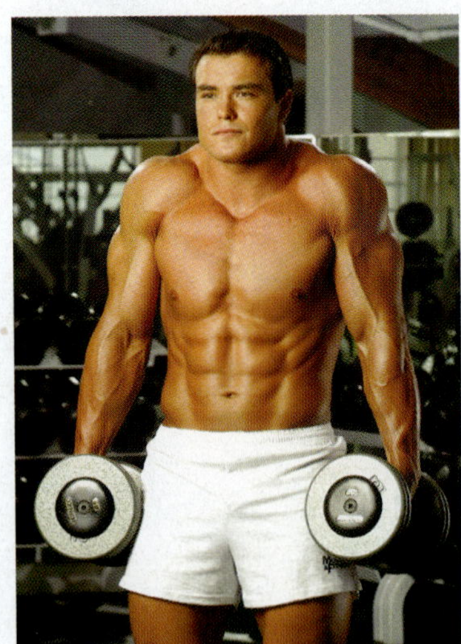

You should restrict shoulder movement to the up-and-down plane.

49

THE SHRUG

Should I rotate my shoulders in a circular fashion as I do dumbbell shoulder shrugs? This would seem to work the traps in a number of angles.

A: The value of any exercise is determined by how effectively it strengthens the movement pattern the muscle in question is designed for. The function of the traps is fourfold:
- Elevation of the shoulder blades;
- Upward turn of the shoulder blades;
- Downward turn of the shoulder blades;
- Retraction of the shoulder blades.

Thus, simply raising the shoulders upward will develop stronger traps. Rotating your shoulders in a circular fashion, however, increases the risk of injury because this type of motion isn't completely natural for this joint. In addition, doing the shrug with weights in your hands increases the potential of pulling the ball joint of the shoulder out of the socket slightly, stressing the connective tissues (ligaments and tendons) and, in a sense, loosening the stability of the joint. Naturally, this can adversely affect your strength in other exercises like the bench press and increase the likelihood of shoulder destabilization and possibly dislocation.

Train the traps by simply lifting the shoulders in the up-and-down plane as high as possible. In an effort to engage different areas of the fibers, execute the movement while lying on an incline bench and vary the degree of the incline. Other movements that will stress your traps include power cleans, hang cleans, high pulls, snatches, hang snatches, deadlifts and upright rows.

50

TRIPLE PRESS

What's the difference between performing triceps pressdowns with an overhand vs. an underhand (reverse) grip?

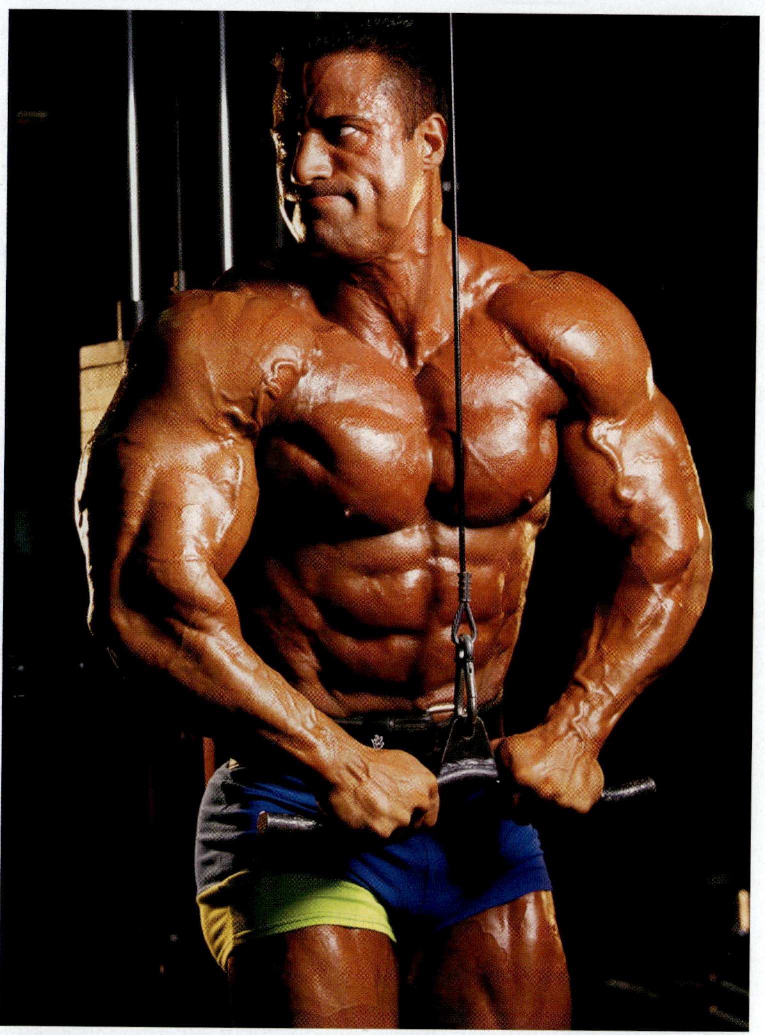

Performing pressdowns with an overhand grip stresses the lateral head.

A: Modifying your grip on the pressdown changes the involvement of the triceps muscle and affects the amount of weight you can use. To better understand this concept, let's take a closer look at this massive upper-arm muscle.

Three Muscles In One

As the name implies, the triceps is composed of three heads — the long head, the lateral (outer) head and the medial (inner) head. At the upper

111

end of the arm, the long head attaches to the scapula (shoulder blade), the lateral head attaches to the upper half of the humerus (upper arm bone) and the medial head attaches to the lower half of the humerus. The muscle fibers of each head run down the back of the arm to converge on one common tendon that crosses the elbow joint and attaches on the ulna (forearm bone). All three heads work in unison to perform the same function — extension of the forearm. In addition, the long head works to extend the upper arm at the shoulder joint, such as during pullovers.

Angle of Attack

Due to their common attachment near the elbow, the three heads of the triceps cannot be isolated during pressdowns. The emphasis can be slightly shifted from one head to another by altering the movement or the angle at which you perform the exercise. Altering your grip changes the angle of stress, modifying muscle involvement and activation.

An overhand grip places the greatest stress on the lateral head, the largest and most prominent part of the triceps muscle. This grip also permits the use of greater weight due to

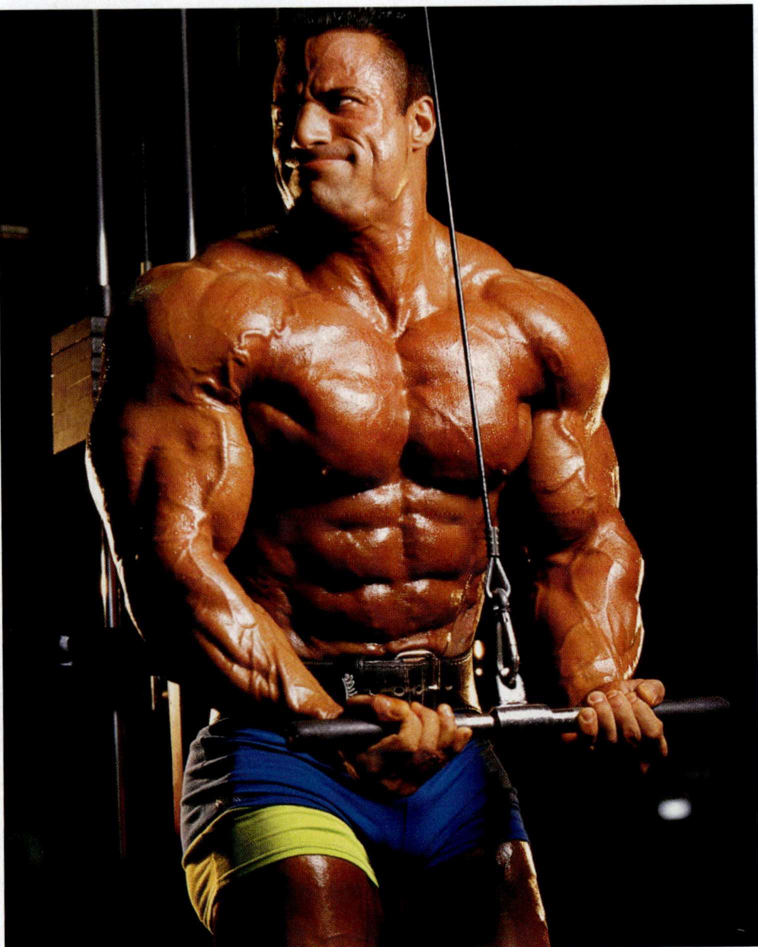

An underhand grip stresses the medial head, forcing the triceps to work alone.

involvement of the chest and shoulder muscles. Although triceps isolation is reduced, the added resistance can result in greater mass if you observe proper form and execution.

Using an underhand grip shifts more emphasis to the medial head of the triceps. Contribution from assisting muscles is virtually eliminated, so you won't be able to use much weight. That's why the reverse-grip pressdown is an excellent isolation exercise that channels all force directly to the triceps.

Optimal Blend

Because the overhand- and underhand-grip pressdown

each offers unique benefits, rotate both through your triceps routine to ensure even development. Do overhand pressdowns early in your triceps workout as a mass-builder. Reserve reverse-grip pressdowns for the end of the workout to isolate the triceps with a final burn.

51

TARGETING TRI'S

My lateral triceps lack in comparison to my long head as well as medial part. Which exercises target this region the most?

A: Any exercise that extends your elbow will work all three heads of your triceps; this is basic anatomy. While you simply can't isolate one part of any muscle over another with different exercises, the triceps is somewhat unique in that it has three distinct heads. Not only that, but the long head's attachments are such that this part of your triceps is recruited slightly more than the lateral and medial heads in movements where your elbows are over your head. Examples are the overhead triceps extension and the french press, if you allow the dumbbells, barbell or EZ-bar to extend beyond your head. Conversely, any exercise that keeps your upper arms to your sides — such as pressdowns, reverse pressdowns and one-arm cable pressdowns — or at 90 degrees to your upper body, such as close-grip benches, will hit the medial and short heads slightly more. This means you can slightly emphasize one area over another, but the medial and short heads are always crankin' irrespective of the exercise.

So here are more questions: Can the slightly greater amount of emphasis found in over-the-head exercises add up to significantly greater long-head growth patterns? If you skipped those exercises, would you get more development in the short and medial heads than in the long head? Frankly, we don't have the answers, but we're skeptical. What you're basically left with is your unique development in this area; you'd be hard-pressed to change your genetics. But the good news is that this really has no bearing on your ability to grow. Pump some serious iron, focusing on progressively moving heavier and heavier weights.

Try hitting your tri's twice a week. Train them hard and heavy for two weeks straight, then in the third week, go hard

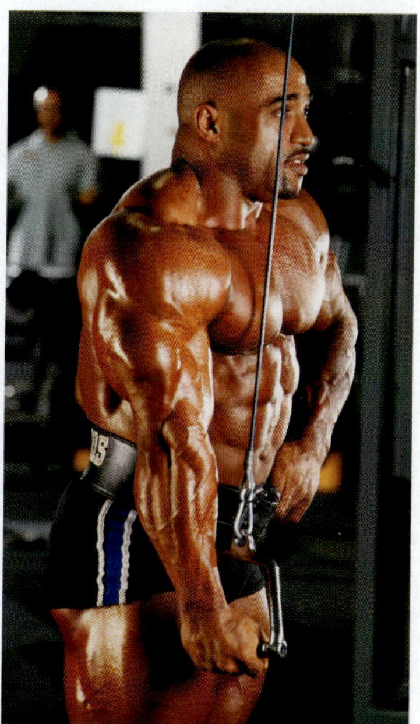
A one-arm cable pressdown hits the medial and short heads hard.

'Don't let the weights dictate your movement; you dictate the movement to the weights. Make your triceps do the work!'

and heavy on the first training day and easy on the second. For the fourth week, go easy on the first day and go to failure on the second. Then repeat the cycle. As you're hitting it hard, though, don't overlook proper technique. Don't let the weights dictate your movement; you dictate the movement to the weights. Make your triceps do the work! Continue to pump away and you'll notice your tri's getting stronger and bigger. With the added size, I bet you'll find that your tri's will take on a more balanced look.

52

DOUBLE DIPPING

I know dips are good for chest and triceps development, but how do I train one without involving the other?

A: Muscle isolation is a misnomer — no matter how hard you try, you just can't completely isolate a given muscle group. Assistant and stabilizer muscles are called upon to some degree in every movement, so even machines designed specifically to isolate fall short of that claim. Nonetheless, shifting the emphasis of some exercises from one muscle group to another is possible, especially in the case of multijoint movements that simultaneously work two or more muscle groups.

The parallel-bar dip is such a compound exercise, working both the triceps and the pectorals via the elbow and shoulder joints, respectively. The body is mostly upright in this dip variation, often with a slight forward lean. The degree of forward lean is a key element in determining whether the dip emphasizes the chest or triceps.

Dips for Triceps

Triceps involvement is greatest when you perform the dip with your body vertical (perpendicular to the floor) and your arms tight to your sides. This reduces movement at the shoulder, restricting it almost entirely to the elbow joint. In this position the triceps contract maximally since they're forced to bear your entire bodyweight (more or less, depending on the apparatus and accessories).

Dips for Chest

Leaning forward and allowing

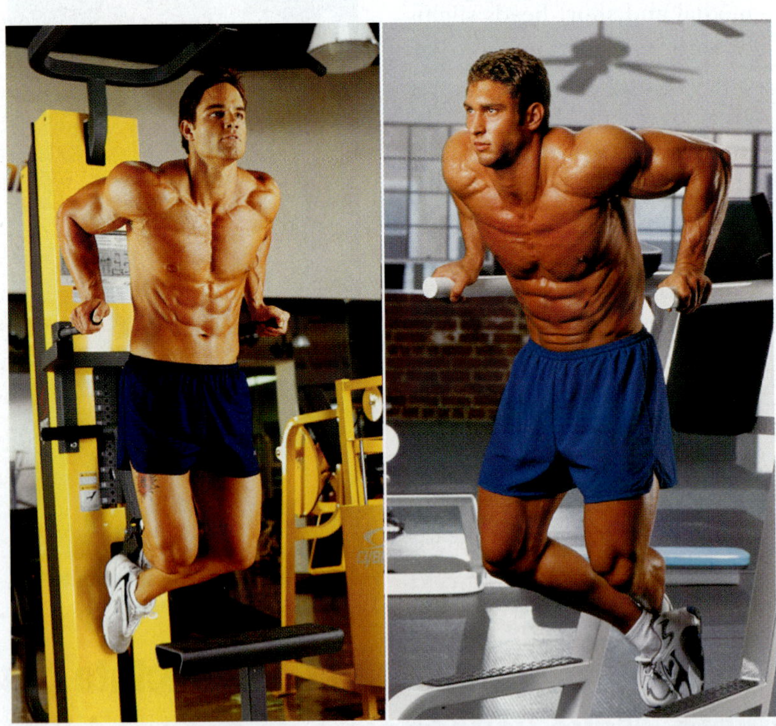

When vertical, the triceps are involved. Leaning forward works the chest harder.

your arms to flare out a bit shifts more of the dip's emphasis from the triceps to the chest. Your chest is involved to a greater degree as your forward lean increases. Of course, strength and balance become an issue as the forward lean becomes excessive, so lean only as far forward as is comfortable (probably no more than 35–40 degrees). Allowing your arms to move out and away from your sides increases the amount of adduction (bringing the upper arms back down to the sides of the body), making it easy to see how this increases tension on the pecs. Eliminating the triceps from any chest-pressing movement is impossible, but these changes in biomechanics will reduce the triceps emphasis and help target the chest. ■

Mixing the Dip

Now that you know how to alter your body mechanics in the dip to target the chest or triceps, the next step is learning how to modify the difficulty of the move based on your strength requirements. If you're fairly weak in the dip, check out our Little Dipper tips. If you want to make the dip harder and more effective, regardless of which muscle you're targeting, try the Big Dipper tips.

LITTLE DIPPER

- Perform it first in chest or triceps routine.

- Have a spotter hold your feet and assist as needed.

- Use a Gravitron machine.

- Lift yourself up to the top and do negatives.

- Use a dip machine; you can adjust the weight to considerably less than your bodyweight.

BIG DIPPER

- Perform it last in chest or triceps routine.

- Perform it second in a compound set.

- Use a weight chain belt to add weight.

- Accentuate the negative by lowering on a count of 4.

- Use a dip machine; you can adjust the weight to considerably more than your bodyweight.

References

1. Haggmark, T., Thorstensson, A. Fibre types in human abdominal muscles. Acta Physiologica Scandinavica 107(4):319–325, 1979.

2. Clemson, J.M., Aaron, C. Effect of grip width on the myoelectric activity of the prime movers in the bench press. Journal of Strength and Conditioning Research 11(2):82–87, 1997.

3. Barnett, C., Kippers, V., Turner, P. Effects of variations of the bench press exercise on the EMG activity of five shoulder muscles. Journal of Strength and Conditioning Research 9(4):222–227, 1995.

4. Simpson, S.R., et al. Comparison of one repetition maximum between free weight and Universal machine exercises. Journal of Strength and Conditioning Research 11(2):103–106, 1997.

5. Rubin, M.R., et al. Effects of free weight vs. machine bench press training on strength development. 1998 NSCA Free Communications: Research.

6. Chilibeck, P., et al. A comparison of strength and muscle mass increases during resistance training in young women. European Journal of Applied Physiology 77:170–175, 1998.

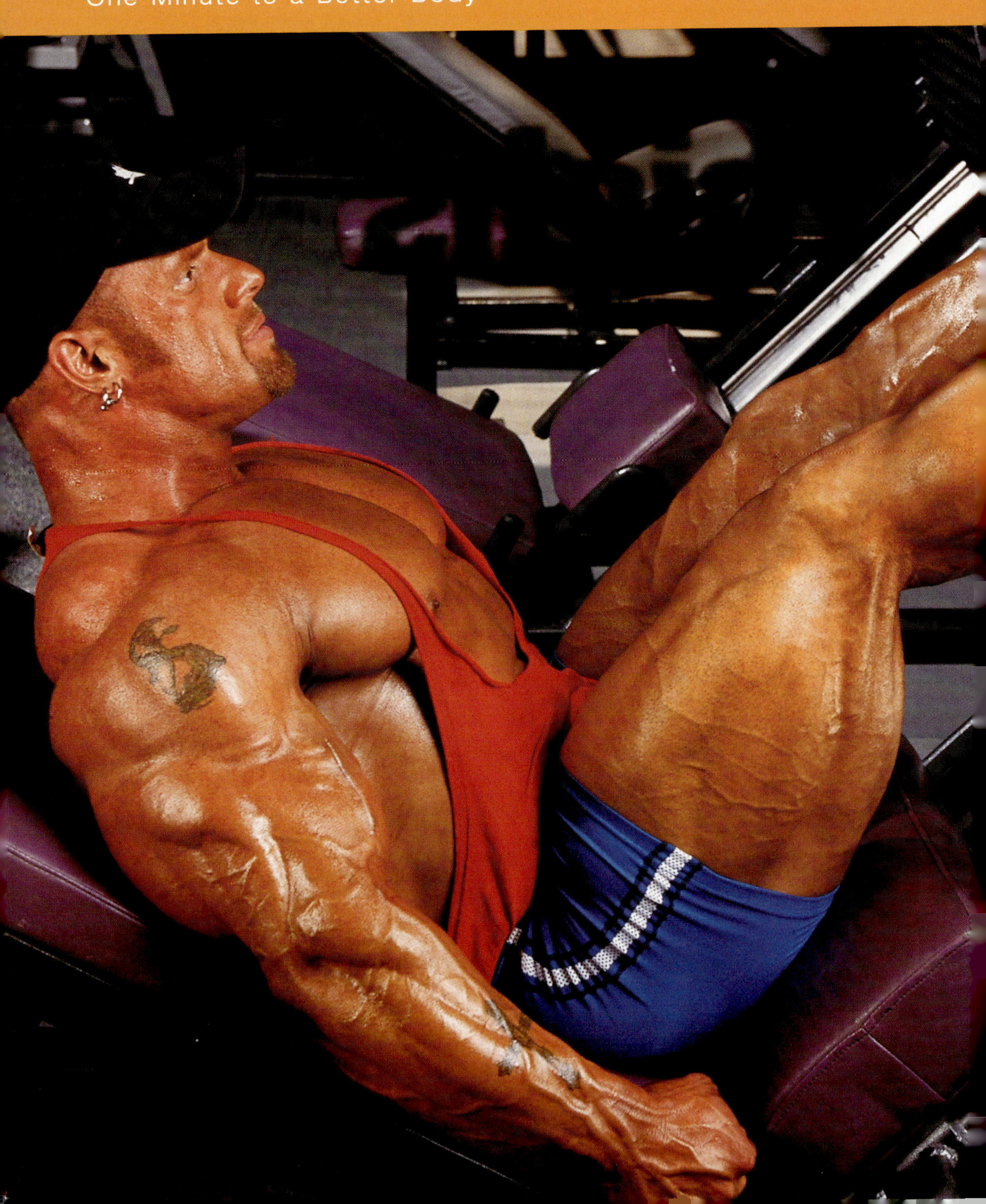

STEEL WHEELS

Exercise techniques and tips to beef up your legs

We see them every time we go to the gym: Guys with pumped, primed upper bodies — and legs so slim they make Heidi Klum jealous. That's not you, of course. Still, it's important to remember that while massive pecs and biceps are worth pursuing, ignoring your legs for too long makes your body look a little off-balance. Not good.

Fortunately, this section's designed to keep that from happening. We've done all the legwork to answer your pressing questions: How deep should you go on squats? What's the difference between standing and seated calf raises? What are the benefits of single-leg training? Should you train your hips? Yup, it's all here. We'll leave the heavy lifting to you.

But before we dive into specifics, here are some general leg-training tips. Keep these in mind while you're honing a lower body your upper body can be proud of.

117

Warm up. Stretch and do a couple of warm-ups before taking on really heavy weight.

Complete the movement. For growth, you've got to go through the full range of motion on every rep of every exercise. Complete movements with slightly lighter weights will take you much farther than sloppy, partial movements with heavy weights. Remember: Partial movements equal partial development.

Remember your form on the positive and negative. On the positive part of the motion, try not to bounce or jerk to get the weight up. And to maximize every rep, don't relax on the negative part; lower the weight with a slow, even motion.

Don't lock out. Even when you're tired, avoid locking out on squats and leg presses. Doing so shifts the stress from the muscle to the knee joint, decreasing muscle-fiber recruitment while increasing risk of injury.

Train your weaknesses as well as your strengths. Otherwise, disparities in strength and size will only grow. Not only can this look funny, but the imbalance can increase your risk of injury as well. For example, research shows that many hamstring injuries are the result of overdeveloped quads and underdeveloped hams. Don't let that be you.

Finally, variety is the spice of leg work. Because legs are such a large, dense muscle group, you need to hit them with a lot of sets, and from a lot of angles, to properly work them. Vary both your exercises and your foot positions within exercises so as to continually challenge your muscles and force them to grow.

Steel Wheels: Questions and Answers

TO SQUAT OR NOT TO SQUAT

It seems that almost all the champs agree that squats are a must for optimal quad development. I do squats in just about every leg workout, but over the last couple of weeks I've found it difficult to get into them. I was wondering, is it really necessary to squat all the time?

A: The reason most successful bodybuilders, and actually athletes in just about any sport, consider the squat an excellent exercise is because it involves nearly all of the muscles in your thighs, your calves for balance and your back muscles as they keep you upright. If you really end up pushing the envelope in terms of how many reps you do in each set, you'll find that your cardiovascular system is

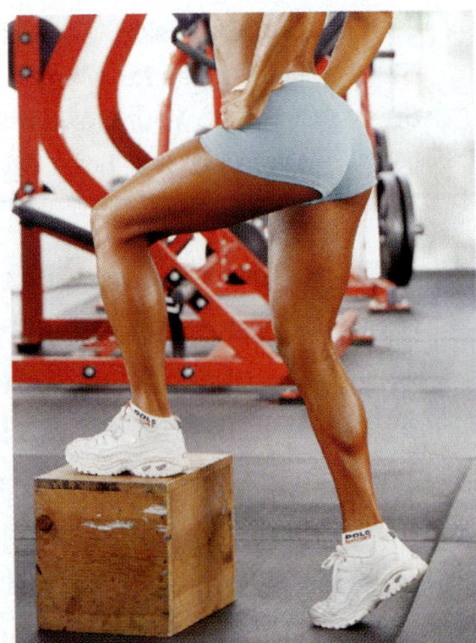

Step-ups are an effective exercise to add variety to a leg workout.

immensely stressed as well. Of course, another cool part of the squat is that its effectiveness is supported by a great deal of research.

Now, to answer your question specifically, no. In fact, your loss of desire to squat may be an indication that your training is getting stale, and this lack of motivation may actually translate into less-effective workouts for other muscle groups, too. If this is the case, you won't be able to expect much to happen in the gains department. A change is in order!

One way to avoid this stalemate is to simply reduce your sets and reps as well as the intensity of your squats. If this isn't enough, try some other exercises that work your thighs in a similarly effective manner, thus reducing the frequency of squatting. Consider doing step-ups, one-legged squats off a bench and lunges. If these exercises are still too demanding and you have a hard time seeing them through, look at some of the physically less-demanding exercises such as leg extensions and leg presses.

Go ahead — do something different for a while and pick up squats when you're fresh in mind and body.

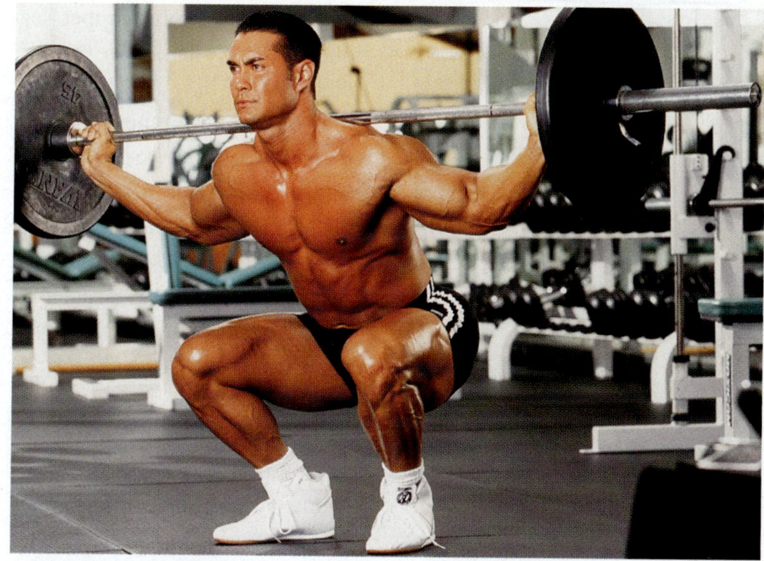

Taller lifters might limit downward motion to avoid knee and back problems.

54

A QUESTION OF DEPTH

I've always heard that I should squat until my thighs are parallel to the ground, but I see others squat lower. What's best?

A: The rule of thumb for squatting is to descend until your thighs are parallel to the ground. This guideline works well for the casual lifter, but some bodybuilders will benefit from a deeper squat. Likewise, other bodybuilders will find that a shallower squat suits them best.

Deep squats (lower-than-parallel thighs, or less than 90 degrees of knee flexion) are popular among powerlifters and Olympic lifters — the same lifters who can't wear normal pants because their thighs are so massive. Coincidence? We don't think so. Most likely the muscle development is directly related to the increased range of motion and muscle activity of the deep squats, not to mention the tremendous amount of weight used. But deep squats aren't a guarantee of tree-trunk thighs; in fact, they may

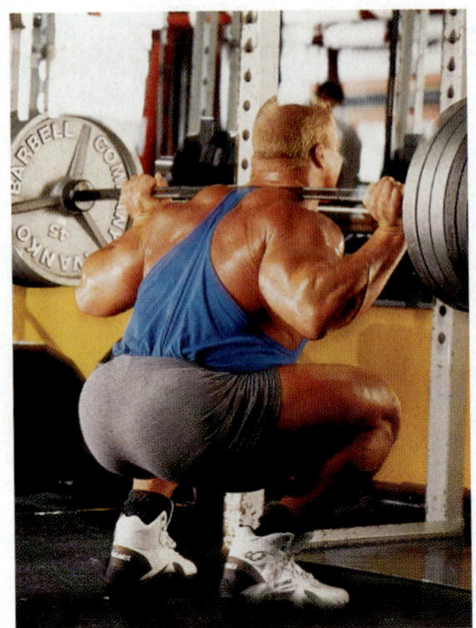

Some bodybuilders descend until their glutes nearly touch the floor.

increase your risk of injury.

No doubt about it, squats place a great deal of stress on the knee joint. Initially, the quad muscles pull the kneecap into the knee joint, providing stability. Yet the compressive forces increase as your body descends, eventually becoming strong enough to cause joint damage in some individuals (especially when performed on a regular basis). Unfortunately, the point at which the risk of injury outweighs the benefits of increased muscle involvement varies from one person to the next. The cutoff has been arbitrarily set at 90 degrees of knee flexion.

Bodytype also determines the depth to which you can squat. Short bodybuilders are able to squat so low their glutes nearly touch the floor. Tall lifters — those with a longer femur (upper leg bone) — simply have more trouble doing so. They have a higher center of gravity, requiring them to bend excessively at the knees and/or waist to keep their balance. This puts even more strain on their knees and lower back, opening the door for more serious problems. Most long-legged lifters are lucky if they can squat to the 90-degree knee position at all.

If you're tall, don't force the issue by performing heavy squats beyond your limits or with bad form. Instead, limit your downward motion and choose different exercises to sculpt your thighs. Take comfort in the fact that shallow squats can be performed with heavier weights. Although deep squats have the advantage of building mass through increased range of motion and muscle-fiber recruitment, shallow squats are safer and will provide good gains with heavier resistance.

If you're predisposed to knee injury or have a known knee condition, deep squats probably aren't for you. Consider squatting just to the parallel-thigh position or as low as you can without knee pain or discomfort. Your body continually provides feedback, so listen to it. Immediate knee pain during squats or chronic soreness afterward is a telltale sign of excessive knee strain. Bodybuilding isn't just about big muscles — it's also about training smart and staying healthy.

55

HEEL ELEVATION

I sometimes see pictures of bodybuilders squatting with plates or a board under their heels. Why do they do this, and does it make a difference in muscular development or strength?

A: Some people use plates under their heels because they expect it to stress their quads more than if their heels were flat on the ground. Yet many lifters are quite inflexible in their ankles, and squatting with a board or plates underneath their heels makes it easier and keeps their heels from popping up as they descend.

In any case, elevating your heels won't result in added growth or help you lift more weight. In fact, the opposite may be true. When your heels are elevated and you go into a deep knee-bend, your knees have to move forward for you to maintain balance. Noted biomechanist, researcher and powerlifter Tom McLaughlin researched the squat extensively and concluded that the most biomechanically sound execution of the movement occurs, in part, when the knees move forward by no more than 11 degrees. This would be hard to maintain with elevated heels, and subsequently you won't get as much out of the movement as you could.

If you have a problem with your heels popping up, simply work on your technique. Be sure to sit back and go to at least parallel to the ground. If you can't achieve this at first, that's okay — just keep working at it. As you grow more familiar with the exercise and become more flexible, you'll be able to squat with perfect technique and experience the growth and strength that comes along with such a terrific movement.

56

LEG EXTENSION MODIFICATIONS

Is it possible to isolate different parts of the quadriceps muscles when doing leg extensions?

A: The seated leg extension is a single-joint movement with little room for modification, yet slight alterations can bring about substantial changes in muscle involvement and development. The importance of variation, no matter how insignificant it may seem, cannot be emphasized enough, especially if you desire continuous and complete muscle growth.

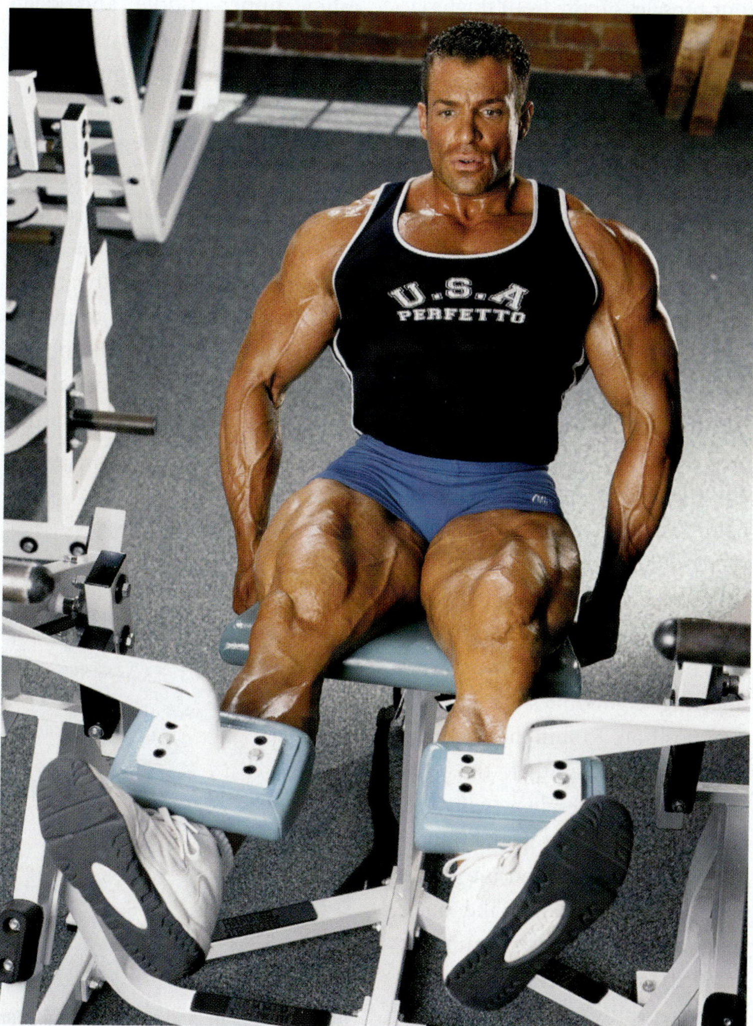

Turning your feet outward on a leg extension emphasizes the inner thighs.

'Performing leg extensions in all three positions ensures that you'll get maximal and symmetrical development in all four quadriceps muscles.'

Extension of the knee (straightening of the lower leg) utilizes all four muscles on the front thigh: 1) rectus femoris (upper-middle), 2) vastus lateralis (outer), 3) vastus medialis (inner) and 4) vastus intermedius (deep). Each muscle is relatively large and all play a significant role in the development of leg strength and mass.

The standard leg extension is the only isolation exercise for the quadriceps. With your feet in the neutral position, toes pointed straight up, the movement stimulates each quad muscle fairly equally. Unless injury or lack of equipment dictates otherwise, this exercise should be a regular part of your leg routine.

The only real modification that can be made without negatively affecting ergonomics or form is foot position. To shift the emphasis of the exercise slightly to the outer thigh (vastus lateralis), turn your feet in. Involvement of the upper-middle and inner quad muscles is reduced slightly while the outer and deep quad muscles assume the majority of the workload. Turning your feet outward does the opposite, transferring the emphasis of the movement to the inner thigh region (vastus medialis). Both the inner, upper-middle and deep quad muscles are maximally stimulated; the outer quad muscle isn't as heavily involved.

With all three leg-extension variations (toes up, toes in and toes out), the deep quad muscle is maximally involved. The vastus intermedius isn't visible in the thigh, but its growth is crucial to overall thigh mass. Development of the deep quad results in a wider, thicker thigh — a more massive foundation for the visible quad muscles to build upon!

Performing leg extensions in all three positions ensures that you'll get maximal and symmetrical development in all four quadriceps muscles. If you have a particularly weak area, you can concentrate your effort on that muscle by performing more of the leg extensions that favor recruitment of that muscle's fibers. For instance, if you lack sweep to your outer quads, perform the majority of your extensions with your toes pointed in. If you lack development in the muscles on the inner side of the knee, then do most sets with your toes pointed out.

As a precaution, experiment with different foot positions using less resistance than you would normally. If you experience joint pain, reduce the degree of foot rotation or revert back to the neutral position. The benefits derived from a modified foot position are quickly erased if it leads to injury.

Small variations may seem trivial in theory and even more insignificant in practice, but your muscles will surely benefit.

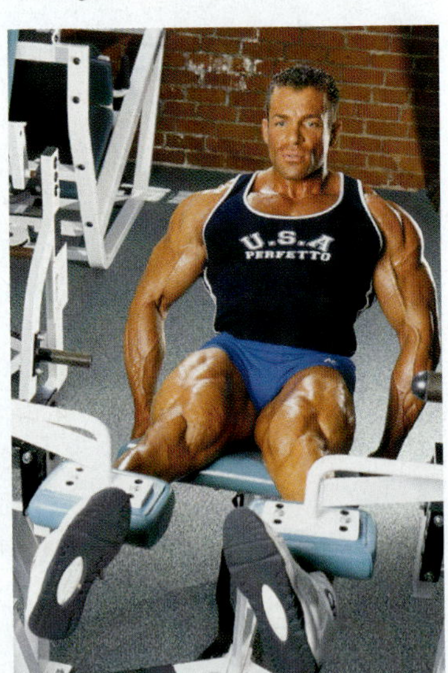

Turn your feet in, and the outer and deep quad muscles assume the workload.

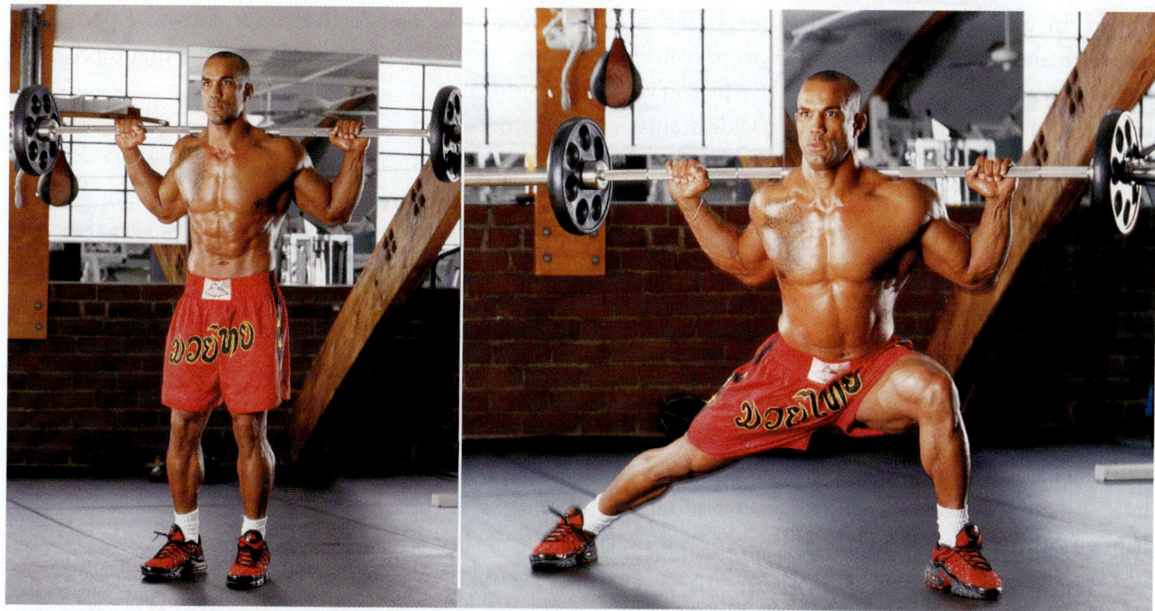

To do a lateral lunge, start with your feet shoulder-width apart (left). Your goal is to lunge completely to the side (right).

A slight modification in muscle-fiber stimulation and motor-unit recruitment is all it takes to keep your muscles off-guard and growing![1]

57

HIP MOVES FOR MEN

Occasionally I see guys on the hip machines doing exercises normally reserved for women. Do these guys know something I don't, or are they simply the sissies they appear to be?

A: No exercise, regardless of how silly or feminine it looks, should be dismissed from the repertoire of a serious bodybuilder. Yes, certain muscle groups — particularly the larger ones — merit greater attention, but none should ever be totally omitted from a training program.

Don't Forget the Small Stuff

Muscle neglect, although not a punishable offense, is certainly a bodybuilding crime. It reduces your potential for maximal development and may increase your risk of injury. Smaller muscles that are never trained outright, even though they contribute during compound movements, will never fully develop, leading to suboptimal size and strength.

The hip muscles are a classic example of a neglected muscle group, especially the hip adductors (inner thigh region). Although not as outwardly visible as the quads or hamstrings, well-developed hip adductors add significant strength and mass to your legs. Similarly, agility and lateral movement are greatly enhanced, and the incidence of groin injury is re-

123

duced in athletes who train their hip adductors.

Even with the guarantee of bigger and stronger legs, you might still be too proud to be seen using the inner thigh machine. If so, don't worry. Other exercises can provide similar — albeit less direct — results.

Modified Squat & Lunge Movements

Both wide-stance squats and lateral (side) lunges work the inner thigh muscles. Use a lighter weight compared to what you normally use with

'Although not as visible as the quads or hamstrings, well-developed hip adductors add significant strength and mass to your legs.'

traditional squats and lunges, because the hip adductors don't require heavy resistance and the knee position of these modified exercises warrants less weight to prevent knee injury.

If you've never performed a wide-stance squat before, start with your feet 6–8 inches wider than your normal squat width and hold a moderately heavy dumbbell between your legs. Experiment with different stance widths, but keep in mind that although hip adductor involvement increases as your stance widens, so does knee strain. Reduce the resistance accordingly.

The lateral lunge carries the same precautions, especially as you step farther to the side. Perform the movement like a regular lunge, but step slightly to the outside instead of straight ahead. At first, an angle of 20–30 degrees is sufficient. As you become more comfortable, widen your step until you are lunging completely to the side (see photo on page 59). The leading foot should still point almost straight ahead (nearly perpendicular to your body) to provide greater inner thigh involvement.

You may be skeptical about inner thigh contribution to overall leg strength, but you'll be surprised at the difference doing hip moves makes, and at how sore you'll feel. Add an inner thigh exercise to your leg routine for 3–4 weeks and you should see or feel a difference in leg size and strength after the first month.

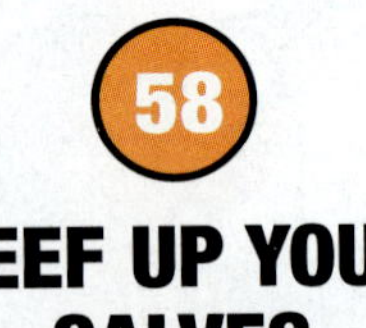

58

BEEF UP YOUR CALVES

Is there any substantial difference between standing and seated calf/heel raises? Do I need to do both, or can I do just one or the other?

A: You'll want to train your calves from both the standing and seated positions if you desire mass and separation. You might think that calf training follows a different set of rules than other muscle groups, but the same principles that build big arms will elicit thick, shapely calves. You've got to hit 'em hard and heavy with a variety of different exercises from as many angles as possible.

The calf region — the muscled area on the back of the lower leg — is composed of several muscles primarily responsible for extension, or plantar flexion, of the foot (movement at the ankle,

'Good gastroc exercises include the standing calf raise, donkey calf raise, or any heel raise/calf press performed on leg-press or hack-squat equipment.'

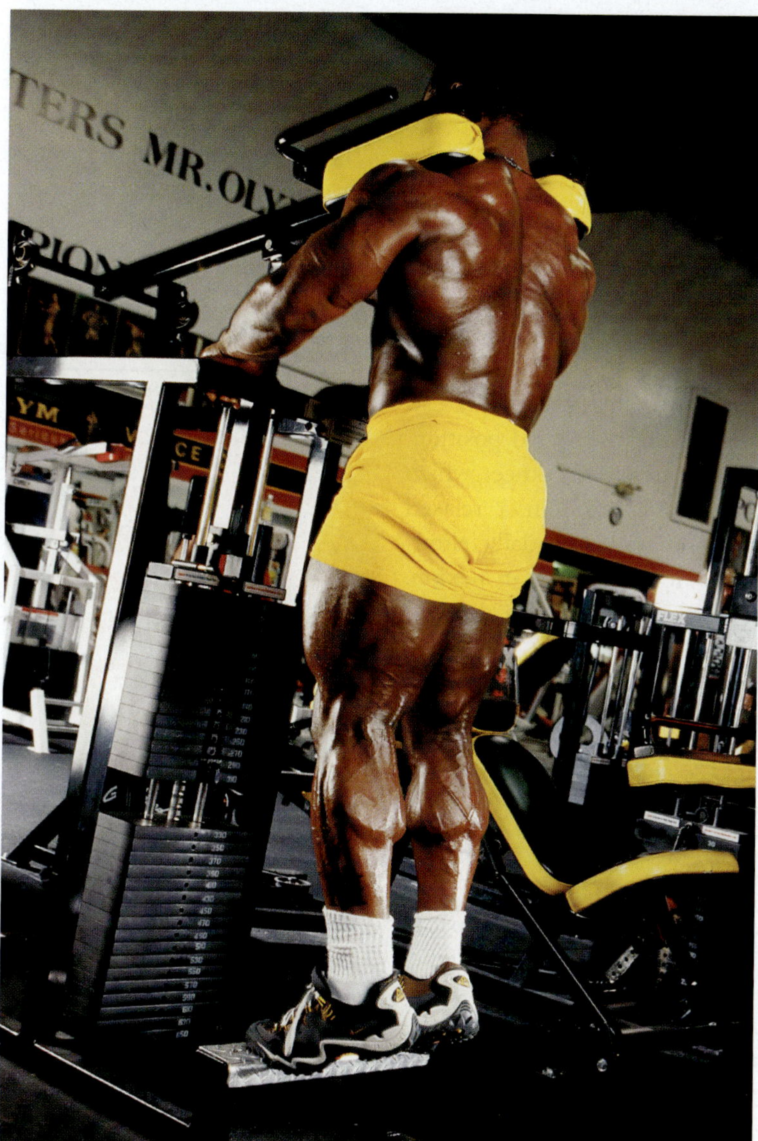

The standing calf raise targets the most predominant calf muscles, the gastrocs.

of the toes away from the body). The most predominant and massive of the calf muscles are the gastrocnemius (gastroc) and soleus. The structure and function of these two muscles necessitate training from both seated and standing positions.

Gastrocs for Width & Shape

The gastroc is the highly visible, diamond-shaped mass of muscle often considered the "calf muscle" itself. Although seen as two distinct heads from the rear, the gastroc is a single muscle. Both heads have a common attachment at the heel (Achilles tendon), but separate attachments at the base of the femur, just above the back of the knee. Because the gastroc crosses the knee joint, it aids in knee flexion. It also means the gastroc contributes little to heel raises performed in the seated position, when the muscle isn't in a stretched position.

To obtain maximal gastroc contraction, the knee must be fully extended, which places the gastroc in a fully stretched position, as when standing. Good

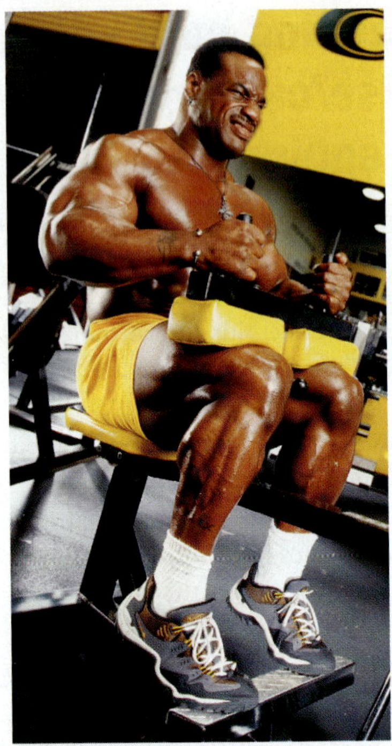

Sitting relaxes the gastroc, and puts the stress of the calf raise on the soleus.

gastroc exercises include the standing calf raise, donkey calf raise, or any variation of heel raises/calf presses performed on leg-press or hack-squat equipment. As the gastroc is the largest and most visible calf muscle from all views, development is essential to ensure continuity between upper and lower leg.

Soleus for Mass & Thickness

The soleus is barely visible on its own, but that doesn't mean it can be ignored. Development will not only add thickness to the calf when viewed from the side but will also add some length, especially at the bottom when viewed from the front or back. The soleus lies almost entirely beneath the gastroc, so even though it can't be seen per se, its presence is certainly noticed when fully developed.

The soleus has the same lower attachment as the gastroc (Achilles tendon), but doesn't cross the knee; its upper attachments are on the upper end of the fibula and tibia (lower leg bones). Complete soleus contraction is achieved with calf raises from the seated position. Sitting flexes the knee, which puts the gastroc in a relaxed position and essentially eliminates it from plantar flexion. Therefore, all stress is diverted to the soleus.

Quick Tips

Much like the abdominals, the calf muscles are resilient and in a perpetual state of contraction, at least when you're on your feet. They're a high-endurance muscle, so you can train them with slightly higher reps (as high as 20), but they'll respond better to moderate reps (6–10) with heavy resistance. Don't be afraid to pile on the weights, as the calves are extremely strong for their size. Additionally, the calves recover quickly; don't allow them to relax, especially at the bottom of the movement. Strive for maximum range of motion with constant tension. At the top, hold the contraction for a second or two as you concentrate on maximally squeezing the working muscle.

ONE LEG AT A TIME

Lately, I've seen a lot of athletes from other sports in the gym working each leg independently during their lower-body training sessions. Will this style of training also benefit bodybuilders?

A: One-legged training has several distinct advantages over training both legs at the same time. Also known as unilateral training, single-limb training allows you to focus on and develop specific muscles without distraction from the other limb. Athletes involved in explosive team sports often use

'Single-leg exercises can reduce gaps between your dominant and non-dominant sides.'

this type of training to improve the strength of their stabilizers, reduce strength imbalances, and improve their strength and power in two-legged lifts.

Of course, the benefits of unilateral training aren't reserved for lower-body muscles alone. You've probably turned many upper-body movements into single-limb exercises by using dumbbells and working one side at a time. Single-leg training, however, is much more difficult. With the exception of lunges or step-ups, it's likely that you've never experienced the following benefits of working each leg independently:

Better Contraction
With only one leg to contend with, you'll find it much easier to visualize and concentrate on the contracting muscle. The result is a better "feel" for the movement and more complete muscle contraction. In fact, research shows that muscle contraction forces are greater when a movement is executed unilaterally compared to bilaterally (both sides).[2]

Improved Symmetry
Unilateral training is perfect for eliminating muscle imbalance and promoting symmetry. It's not uncommon for the same muscle group to be disproportionate from one limb to the other, especially when it comes to legs. If you always train both legs together, your stronger side is forced to handle a greater proportion of the weight as you fatigue, and the gaps in strength and size become larger. Single-leg exercises can reduce these gaps between your dominant and non-dominant sides.

Muscle Shock
Whenever you find a new way to stimulate muscle, you have to jump on it. Single-leg training changes the way you overload

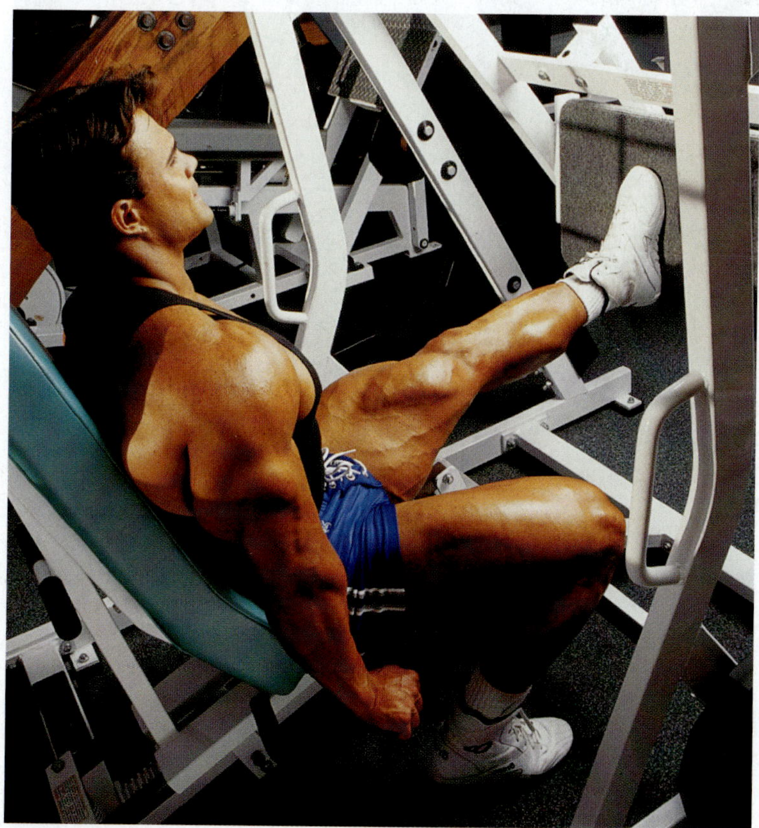

Unilateral, as opposed to bilateral, training allows for better focus, feel and contraction.

stimuli and initiating a new growth phase.

Increased Muscle Involvement

One-legged movements require more support and balance, demanding greater involvement of stabilizer muscles. Developing your stabilizers adds to the overall strength of the muscle group they support. You won't notice it immediately, but you'll be pleasantly surprised when you switch back to two-legged training, only to realize that you're able to handle significantly more weight.

Effective Tool When Injured

Injury is a common byproduct of training, often resulting in considerable downtime. Unilateral training is useful when one limb is injured, allowing continued training of the other. Additionally, many of the strength gains and neural adaptations of the exercising muscle are transferred to the non-exercising muscle of the opposite limb,[3] which can speed recovery.

Increased Calorie Utilization

Training one side at a time means your workouts will take a little longer, but the upside is that you'll burn more calories. You can rest one leg while the other works, so you won't need as much rest between sets (if you

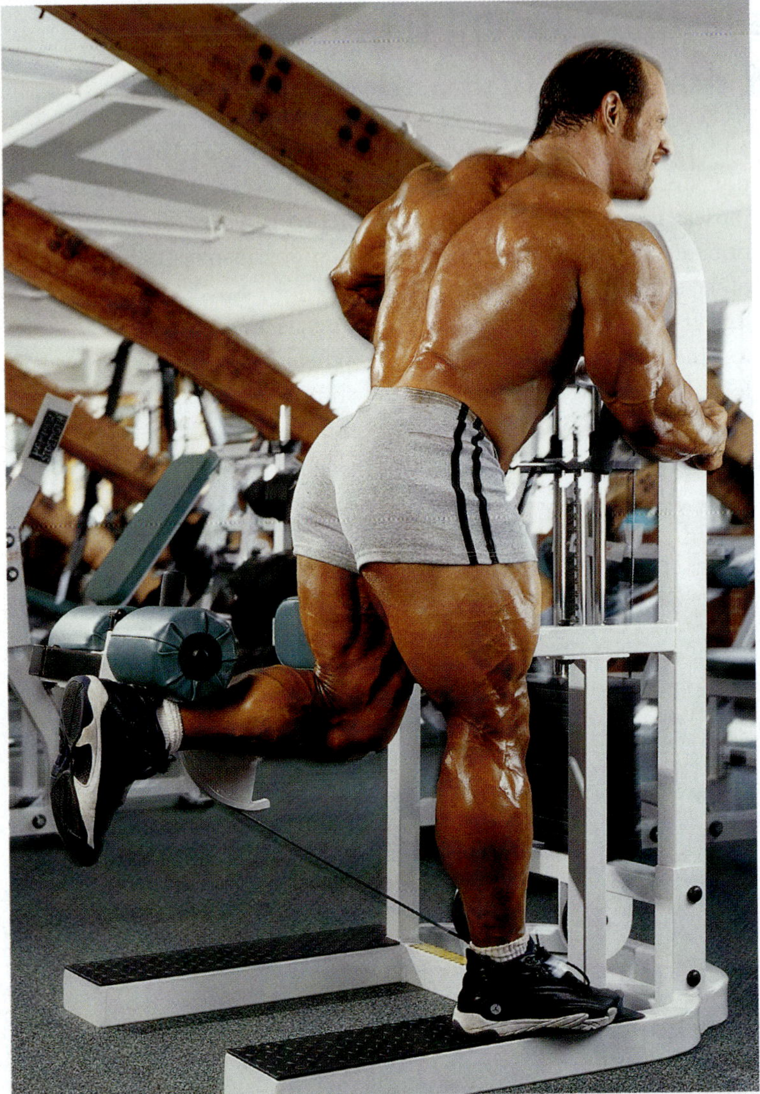

Performing a move with only one leg requires your stabilizer muscles to work harder.

your muscles, forcing them to fire slightly differently to balance the weight. What exactly does that mean? Well, think back to your first few months of weight training. You felt uncoordinated and shaky at times, but what about the incredible gains you made in strength and size? That's what muscle shock is all about — exposing your muscles to fresh alternate legs every set). Each leg will get adequate rest, yet your cardiovascular system will get less. Don't expect big improvements in aerobic conditioning, but you'll do more work with less total rest and burn more calories.

Try substituting one-legged exercises for your regular two-leg lifts for four weeks — squats, presses, curls and extensions. When you return to your regular program, your wheels will be bigger, stronger and more powerful than ever! ■

References

1. Tesch, P.A. Target bodybuilding. Champaign, IL: Human Kinetics, 1999.

2. Archontides, C., Fazey, J.A. Inter-limb interactions and constraints in the expression of maximum force: a review, some implications and suggested underlying mechanisms. Journal of Sports Science 11(2):145–158, 1993.

3. Kannus, P., Alosa, D., Cook, L., et al. Effect of one-legged exercise on strength, power and endurance of the contralateral leg. A randomized, controlled study using isometric and concentric isokinetic training. European Journal of Applied Physiology and Occupational Physiology 64(2):117–126, 1992.

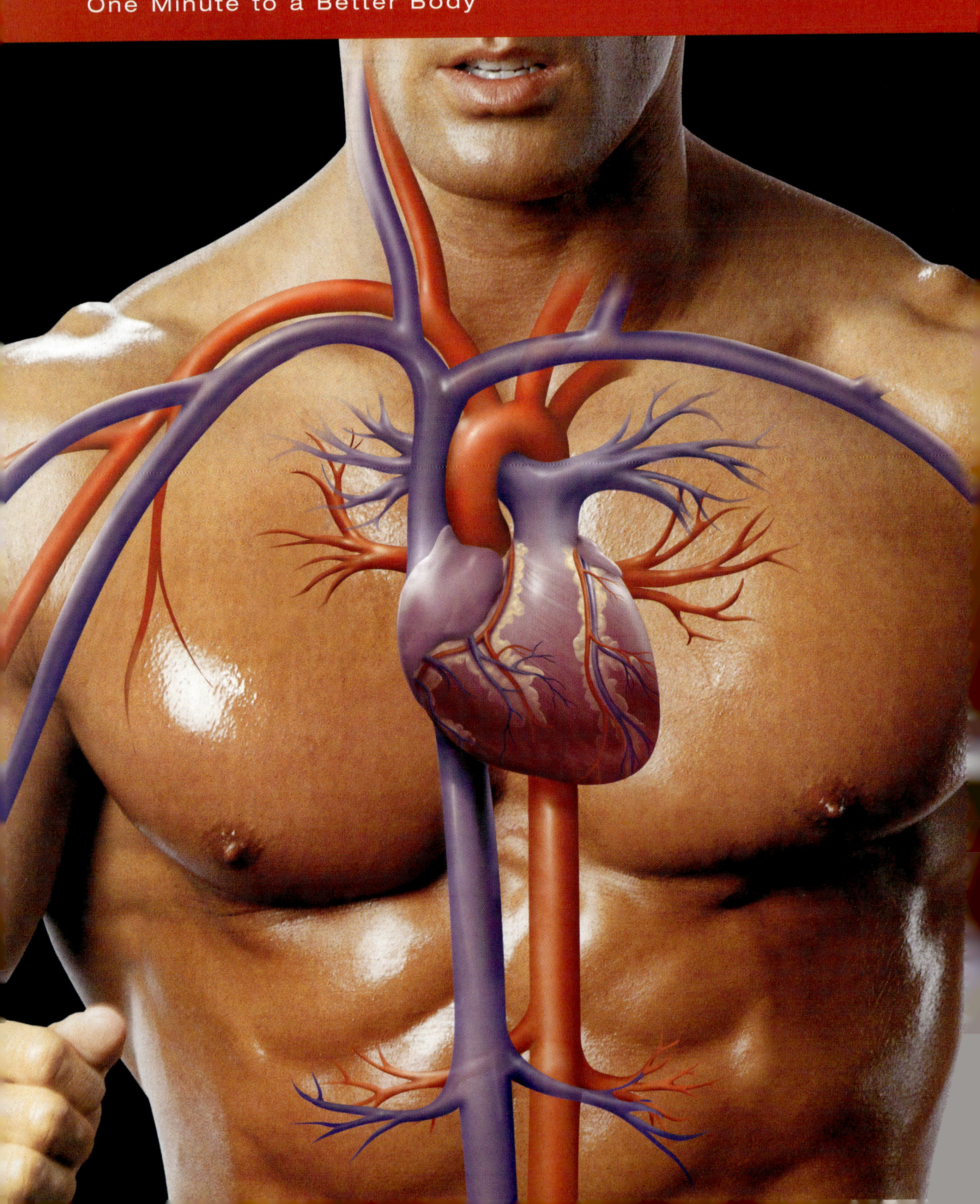

HEART SMARTS

Effective cardio training to dial in your lean physique

You look great, your biceps are swelling and your pecs have almost popped the buttons off your shirt. But you still have a little too much bodyfat obscuring your abs, and when you walk up the stairs to your apartment, you huff and puff. If you have to carry grocery bags loaded with protein powder and canned tuna, you can hardly catch your breath. It's embarrassing.

Even worse, it's unhealthy. Your hard, muscular body belies an out-of-condition cardiovascular system. You can't put off that cardio program any longer. Sure, your real desire is to build muscle, but what good will a great physique do you if you can't get around to enjoy it and show it off? No more excuses that aerobics is for people who can't lift weights. On the contrary, a real aerobic workout will kick your butt to the moon and back.

Maybe you've heard that cardio burns up your hard-earned muscle. Truth is, the relatively small amount of aerobics you need to condition your cardiovascular system won't flatten your muscles. In fact, aerobic activity will burn off fat and unneeded calories, revealing a tighter, leaner and more defined body. Cardio work also boosts metabolism, strengthens your heart and lungs, and lowers your risk of heart disease and certain cancers.

As a bodybuilder, your immediate interests probably include reducing your existing bodyfat and avoiding bodyfat gain. As you become better conditioned, aerobic training will help your cells become better fat-burning furnaces.

Just how much cardiovascular fitness is necessary to reap the maximum benefits? That question isn't so easily answered. Intensity and duration of the workout, your fitness level and genetic makeup are just a few of the influencing factors. But don't fret: You can still get the results you want without making the process an exact science.

Hit the Ground Running

No magic formula can determine the best cardio program for you, but this section will simplify things a bit. With all the variables involved, including your own preferences, you just need to try different activities to see what works. A few guidelines, though, can help you get started in the right direction. Find which body type best describes you to get an idea of where to begin.

Endomorph: For the person who tends to gain and hold bodyfat easily, a challenging but safe cardio workout is a

must. Choose activities that keep jarring of joints and tissues to minimum. Start slowly, 20–30 minutes in duration 3–4 times a week. Gradually increase frequency until you're up to 5–6 days a week, then slowly lengthen the sessions. Work in the lower end of your target heart-rate range until your conditioning improves.

Mesomorph: Being naturally muscular could also mean that you're overweight for your height. Just like the endomorph, you should stay away from aerobic activities that could potentially cause back and joint problems. A good choice is cycling. If you're new to cardio activities, start slowly, working up to 4–5 days a week, 20–30 minutes each session. Depending on your goals, you may wish to cycle the intensity of your workouts for better results.

Ectomorph: A person who is naturally lean probably doesn't have too many problems with walking and running. But just like anyone else, you should find a mode of exercise that's enjoyable. If you're just starting out, keep your cardio sessions between 20–30 minutes 3–4 days a week at moderate intensity. As your aerobic fitness improves, increase the frequency and duration. You don't need to worry about excess

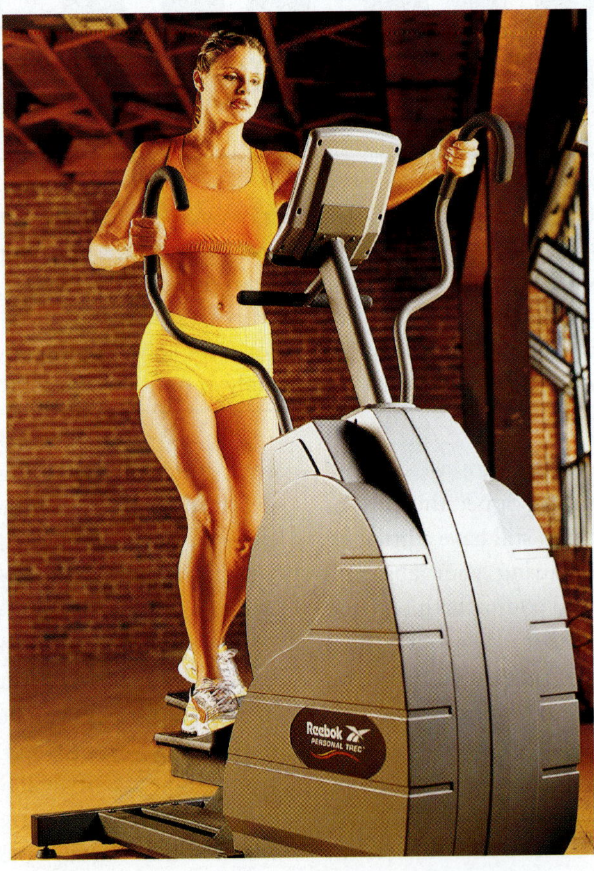

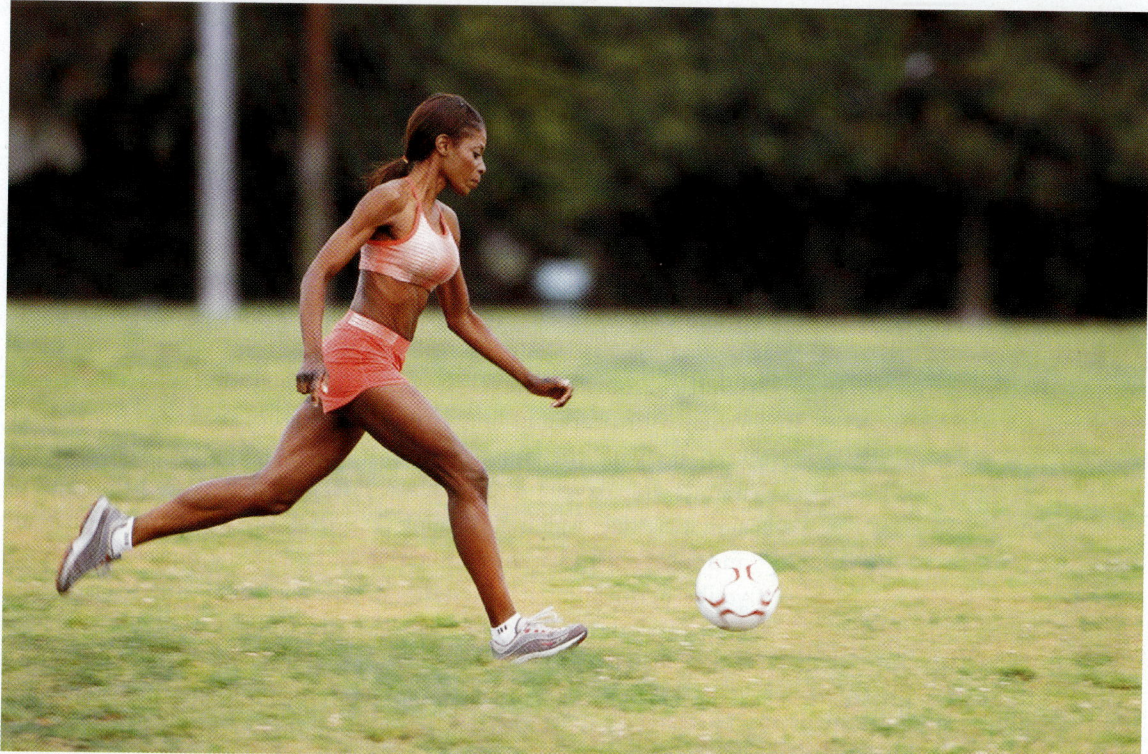

bodyfat, but be careful not to overdo it. Too much cardio could bring you to the point of diminishing returns.

Taking the Next Step: Working Out

Incorporating aerobic work into your already finely tuned program may seem frustrating at best and unbearable at worst. Don't think of it in terms of losing out on valuable lifting time; think of it instead as time devoted to carving out the details of those hard-earned muscles, maximizing recovery time between sets and conditioning your delivery system (heart and lungs) for a higher level of health and fitness.

Plug in the cardio sessions where you're most likely to stick to them.

Increase your workload gradually. For the first few weeks, keep the sessions short and sweet; 15–20 minutes 2–3 times a week.

Choose activities that you really enjoy. (Or, at least avoid the ones you know you hate.)

Record the details of each session (time, length, mode of exercise, how you felt during and after). If at some point you decide to make changes, you can compare the old program with the new.

Don't be afraid to make changes. They will help you discover what works best for you.

On the pages that follow you'll find more helpful tips to advance your cardio training.[1,2]

Heart Smarts: Questions and Answers

60

CARDIO CONFUSION

Should cardio be a part of everyone's routine or just people who are trying to lose weight? And what exactly constitutes a cardio workout?

A: Not all exercise is created equal. The heart requires cardiovascular, or aerobic, exercise for optimum performance gains. Cardio increases the body's ability to carry and utilize oxygen. Bodybuilders need to train their hearts just like anyone else, in spite of their desire to gain freaky physiques. The trick is to do it without burning the muscle mass they've worked so hard to build. This is where nutrition comes in: Eating plenty of carbohydrates and protein will help bodybuilders keep their muscle gains while allowing them to aerobically train their hearts.

Running, walking, jogging, swimming and cycling are examples of aerobic exercise. You don't have to go gung-ho to reap the benefits. Choose an activity you enjoy, begin slowly and be consistent. As your cardiovascular fitness improves, you'll want to increase your exercise intensity and duration.

What's aerobic, anyway?

When your heart and lungs can keep up with the muscles' demands for oxygen created by activities like walking, jogging and non-sprint running, then you're performing aerobic exercise. You can do these activities relatively comfortably because your cardiovascular system is able to provide a steady supply of oxygen to your muscles. When you push yourself beyond your aerobic boundary, you enter the anaerobic zone. In an anaerobic state, your heart and lungs cannot match the demand for oxygen. Going from a jog to a fast sprint will take you there. In anaerobic stages of exercise, instead of using oxygen to burn energy (supplied by glucose and fat), your muscles primarily use forms of quick energy that are stored in the muscle cells. Since these stores don't last long, anaerobic pursuits such as sprinting are of short duration.

Top athletes use anaerobic training to improve their cardio-

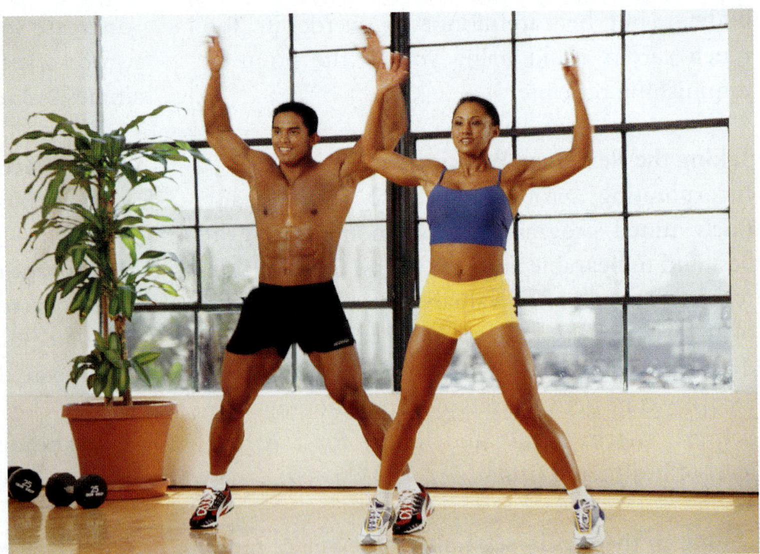

Even five minutes spent doing jumping jacks counts toward your cardio work.

'Bodybuilders need to train their hearts just like anyone else, in spite of their desire to gain freaky physiques.'

vascular endurance and athletic performance. Anaerobic exercise can be used intermittently during an aerobic workout to challenge or overload the cardiovascular system. Such intervals of anaerobic training can increase your aerobic capacity, making subsequent aerobic training feel easier. This method of doing cardio is also believed to enhance fat utilization.

Heart Savings

Consider time spent doing aerobic activities as a type of heart savings: You want to bank at least 30 minutes of aerobic exercise 3–4 times a week to boost your health account. Small contributions add up to big dividends. Five minutes spent walking to the grocery store, 15 minutes doing rigorous housework and 10 minutes enjoying a quick morning walk before work all count.

Exercise within your target heart-rate zone

To find your target heart rate (number of heartbeats per minute), subtract your age from 220. Multiply that number by 0.50 to get the low-end number, then multiply the same number by 0.75

to get the higher number. To measure your pulse, place the fingertips of the index and middle fingers of your right hand on your left wrist

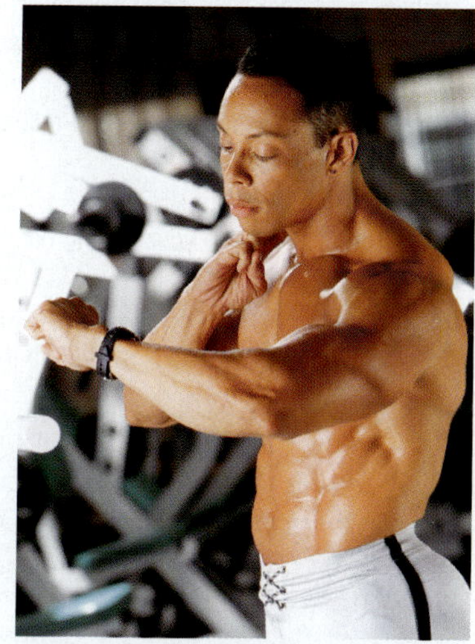

Check your heart rate to make sure you're working within your zone.

between the wrist bone and tendon on the thumb side (palm up). Using a watch with a second hand, start counting the beats when the second hand is at 12. Count beats for 10 seconds and multiply by six. Beginners should start out at the lower end of their target heart-rate training zone; better-conditioned athletes can push themselves harder and work out at a higher heart rate. The benefits of consistent aerobic exercise are that you can burn more total calories and more calo-

ries from fat, plus improve your cardiovascular fitness, as you push yourself harder or longer.

Some people overdo cardiovascular training. Signs that you should stop your workout include difficulty breathing (not just breathing hard), an inability to recover easy breathing shortly after a workout, and pain in the extremities or in the chest. If you experience tightness in your chest during exertion, see your physician.

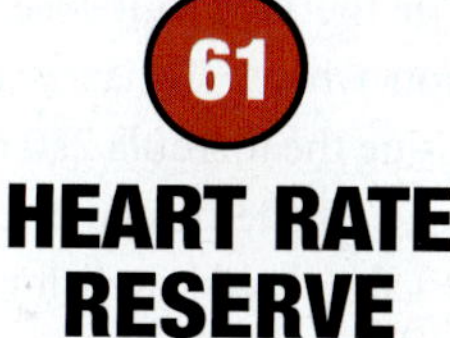

61

HEART RATE RESERVE

A: Several methods exist for determining target heart-rate (THR) range. The method you speak of is likely the Karvonen, or heart-rate reserve method. It's as practical as the traditional technique yet provides slightly more personalized feedback.

Determining THR range can be done directly, by measuring maximal oxygen consumption (VO2 max) in the laboratory, or indirectly, by using formulas based on your maximum heart rate (HRmax). The indirect methods are reliable when HRmax is measured (in the lab), but lose some precision when HRmax is calculated using the formula 220 minus your age. Nonetheless, the estimated value works well for most healthy individuals.

The first indirect method — the traditional and most widely used method — for determining THR involves finding your lower and upper limits (typically 70% and 90%, respectively) of your HRmax. The second indirect method, the Karvonen method, is similar to the first but takes into account your resting heart rate. Including resting heart rate in the equation modifies the THR limits, compensating for individual differences in heart rate and level of cardiovascular fitness. Thus, as you build cardiovascular fitness, your THR increases proportionately.

The lower and upper training limits of the Karvonen method are typically 60%–85%, but are a percentage of heart-rate reserve (HRR), not HRmax. Heart-rate reserve is calculated by subtracting resting heart rate from HRmax. With the Karvonen method, 60%–85% of HRR cor-

---

Karvonen formula

To find your target heart-rate (THR) range using the Karvonen method, you must know your maximum heart rate (HRmax) and your resting heart rate. Then follow these steps:

1) Calculate heart rate reserve (HRR) by subtracting your resting heart rate in beats per minute from your HRmax (220 minus your age).

2) Lower limit:
   a) Take 60% of your HHR.
   b) Add this value to your resting heart rate.

3) Upper limit:
   a) Take 85% of your HHR.
   b) Add this value to your resting heart rate.

Example

This compares the two indirect methods of calculating THR for a 30-year-old individual with a resting heart rate of 65 bpm:

TRADITIONAL	KARVONEN
	(resting HR = 65 bpm per self-measure)
HRmax = 220 − age	HRmax = 220 − age
HRmax = 220 − 30	HRmax = 220 − 30
HRmax = 190 bpm	HRmax = 190 bpm
	HRR = HRmax − resting HR
	HRR = 190 bpm − 65 bpm
	HRR = 125 bpm
Lower HR limit = 70% x HRmax	Lower HR limit = (60% x HHR) + resting HR
Lower HR limit = 0.7 x 190 bpm	Lower HR limit = (0.6 x 125 bpm) + 65 bpm
Lower HR limit = 133 bpm	Lower HR limit =140 bpm
Upper HR limit = 90% x 190 bpm	Upper HR limit = (85% x HHR) + resting HR
Upper HR limit = 0.9 x 190 bpm	Upper HR limit = (0.85 x 125 bpm) + 65 bpm
Upper HR limit = 171 bpm	Upper HR limit = 172 bpm
THR range = 133–171 bpm	THR range = 140–172 bpm

responds to about 70%–90% of HRmax determined by the traditional method.[3]

The THR limits for the two indirect methods are sometimes similar and sometimes not. Both methods provide healthy training zones, but the Karvonen method is preferred because it incorporates more personal data into the formula. Use your THR range along with other indicators, such as breathing rate and perceived exertion, to get the most benefit from your training.

62

DROP ZONE

I've burned a great deal of bodyfat by adding regular cardio sessions to my training, but am having trouble losing that last amount of bodyfat. Would incorporating interval training allow me to increase my intensity and number of calories burned in the same time?

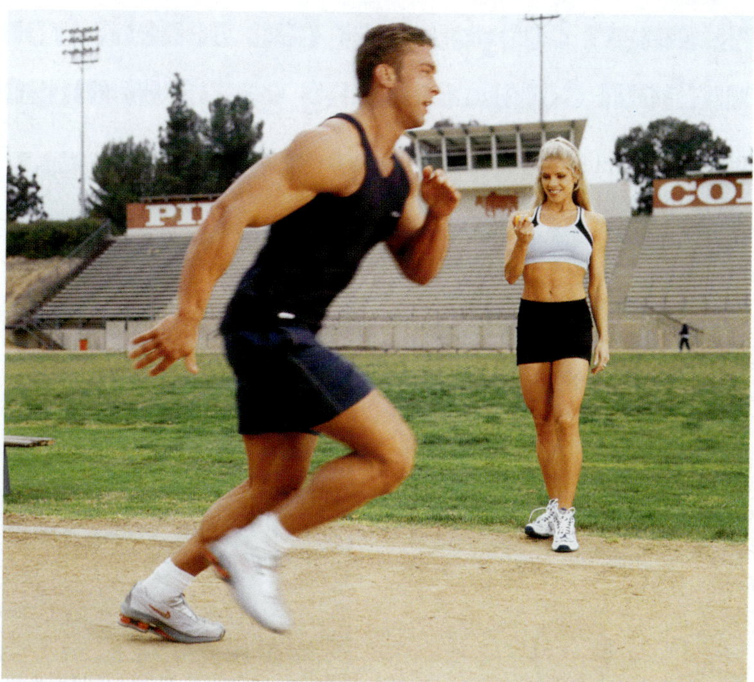

To incorporate intervals into your routine, sprint, then jog at a lower intensity.

A: You'll burn significantly more calories using intervals, meaning your intensity is going to be cycled each time rather than flat-lined across your workout. Interval training is basically alternating periods of intense activity with periods of "working rest," where you're still moving but at a lesser intensity than the actual interval. Warm up five minutes on the machine you're going to use, then do anywhere from 4–8 intervals depending on your ability level. The intervals should be pretty hard, and should last only about 30–60 seconds. Follow each one with about two minutes of moderately paced working rest. Cool down for five minutes to bring your heart rate safely down, then stretch. The whole routine should take about 25–40 minutes total, so it's also great if you're short on time. You can also do intervals outdoors. Try jogging a block or two, then pick something — a car, a tree, a signpost — and sprint to it, then come back to a jog until you recover, and repeat the process.

'A smart bodybuilder can benefit from aerobic training without compromising gains in muscle growth.'

It's About Time

With intervals you're doing the same amount of work time-wise but burning more calories. Intervals, however, can really kick your butt so try doing them no more than three times a week. Allow at least two full days of rest between sessions to fully recover. On the other days, you can do 30–60 minutes of moderate, steady-state cardio.

63

TOO MUCH CARDIO

I'm serious about bodybuilding and want to include cardio in my workouts, but I'm afraid that aerobic training will limit my muscle growth. How much is too much?

A: The debate between mass development and cardiovascular conditioning is long-standing. In the

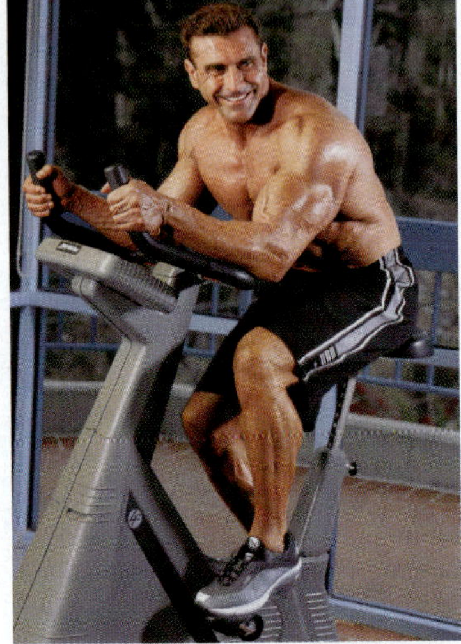

Cardio exercise strengthens your heart and draws upon fat stores.

sport of bodybuilding, cardio is the double-edged sword that burns bodyfat yet simultaneously threatens to deplete hard-earned muscles of their protein content. Although some give and take can exist when the two are combined, a smart bodybuilder can reap the benefits of aerobic training without compromising gains in muscle growth.

Cardiovascular conditioning, or aerobic activity, strengthens the heart and enhances the body's ability to deliver oxygen and nutrients to muscles. Maintaining a healthy cardiovascular system reduces the risks of heart disease and conditions associated with obesity. Aerobic activity also draws upon fat stores, especially when performed at low to moderate levels (80% or less of maximal heart rate).

The benefits of aerobic training speak volumes, but the belief that cardio consumes muscle protein has caused many bodybuilders to limit or even cease cardio training altogether. During aerobic activity, small amounts of protein can be utilized as energy, though the misconception that it significantly depletes muscle stores relates more directly to poor dietary habits.

Dieters who commonly go overboard with aerobic activity don't realize that a good portion of their weight reduction may be due to muscle loss. Muscle protein becomes a chief source of fuel when caloric intake is inadequate. When the body doesn't get enough energy (calories consumed), it must draw upon stored reserves, mainly in the form of fat but also from protein, most of which is found in muscle.

That being said, it's evident

why dieters tend to lose muscle and why bodybuilders shouldn't fear aerobic training. The only real time for concern is before competition, when caloric intake is restricted and aerobic activity is increased. Resistance training during this period will aid in continued muscle protein synthesis, and losses can be further offset with higher protein consumption.

Thirty minutes of moderate-intensity aerobic activity performed most days — preferably every day — is recommended for cardiovascular health benefits.[4] Although this may seem like a lot, it doesn't all have to be performed at one time. Fifteen minutes of cardio before a workout for warm-up and 15 minutes afterward to get fresh blood to the muscles and help remove byproducts of anaerobic metabolism is just one example of the endless cardio combinations you can incorporate into your workouts. Regular aerobic activity need not impede muscle growth if you weight train and eat right. Remember, bodybuilding isn't just about building bigger muscles, it's also about building a better, healthier physique.

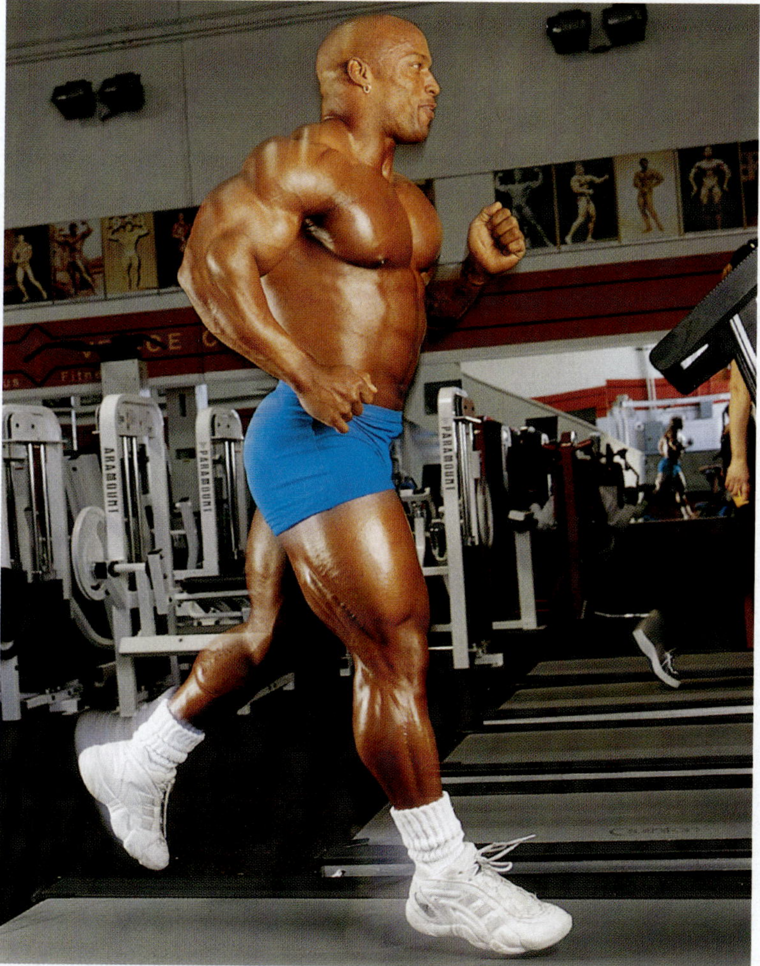

Your heart will reap health rewards from just 30 minutes of cardio each day.

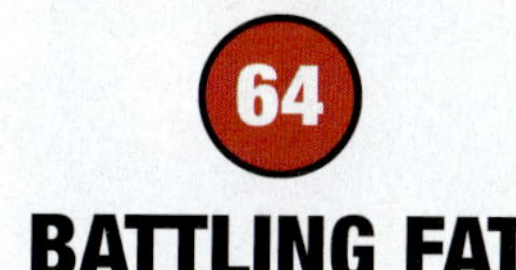

64

BATTLING FAT

Should I do cardio before or after my lightweight bodybuilding, and for how long? Usually I spend two hours doing free weights.

A: It depends on your specific goals. We'll assume you want to get fitter and leaner, build some muscle and increase your strength and

'If you lift with high intensity and engage in intense endurance training as well, your strength, power and size will more than likely be compromised.'

endurance. We'll also assume that you aren't hoping to become an elite athlete in either an endurance or strength sport

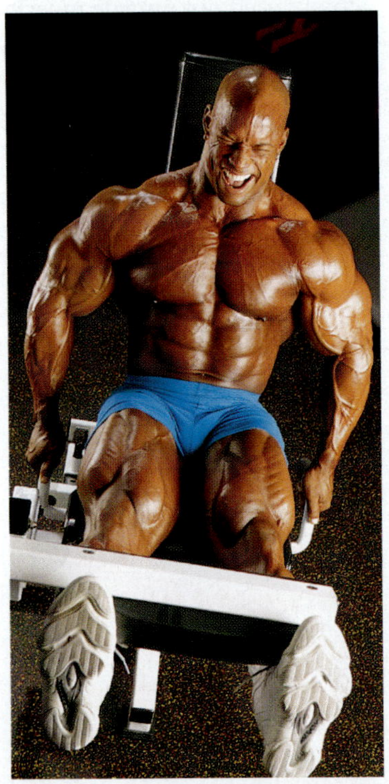

Research suggests you should do weight training before cardio.

nor looking for extreme changes in appearance. We'll guess, too, that you're asking this question because you're after maximal fat control; in other words, would it make a difference to do aerobics before bodybuilding or vice versa in your quest to get as lean as possible?

If this is indeed your situation, the 1998 American College of Sports Medicine's annual conference presented research from Truman State University in Kirksville, Missouri, that has your name written all over it. Researchers recruited nine men and seven women for their study, all of whom were fairly well trained. One group did a 20-minute treadmill workout at 60%–70% of their maximal oxygen uptake (VO2 max) while the other followed the same aerobic training protocol but after lifting weights. The latter consisted of a six-exercise circuit with weights the subjects could handle for 10–12 reps maximally and going to failure on each station.

After reviewing the data, the researchers found that the group that pumped iron first had higher heart rates and lower respiratory exchange ratios — a complicated method that allows exercise physiologists to determine whether the fuel for exercise primarily comes from carbs or fat. The lower the respiratory exchange ratio, the more fat is used to fuel activity. With higher heart rates and lower respiratory exchange ratios, those study subjects who pumped iron before they did aerobics used more bodyfat as fuel than the other group.

In the long term, then, you might reap greater benefits from lifting before you do cardio. You may consider dropping the weights to 60–90 minutes per session and adding about 30 minutes of aerobics. To keep things interesting, vary your intensity between type of exercise and training days. But here we need to address your goals again. Keep in mind that in many respects, aerobics and lifting are polar opposites. If you lift with high intensity and engage in intense endurance training as well, your strength, power and size will more than likely be compromised. Also realize that you can't attain maximal development in either aerobic or anaerobic abilities if you train both with high intensity. As you can see, your goals will strongly influence how you should train.

65

THE HEAT IS ON

I live in Miami and while I love the weather for going to the beach, it makes it nearly unbearable for my runs. I often get a headache or feel weak early into my cardio routine, sweat buckets and seem to overheat. Is there anything I can do to prevent this from happening?

A: Nothing makes you want to bike, run or hike outdoors more than balmy weather. But exercising regularly during the heat of summer brings an increased risk of dehydration, which can lead to other

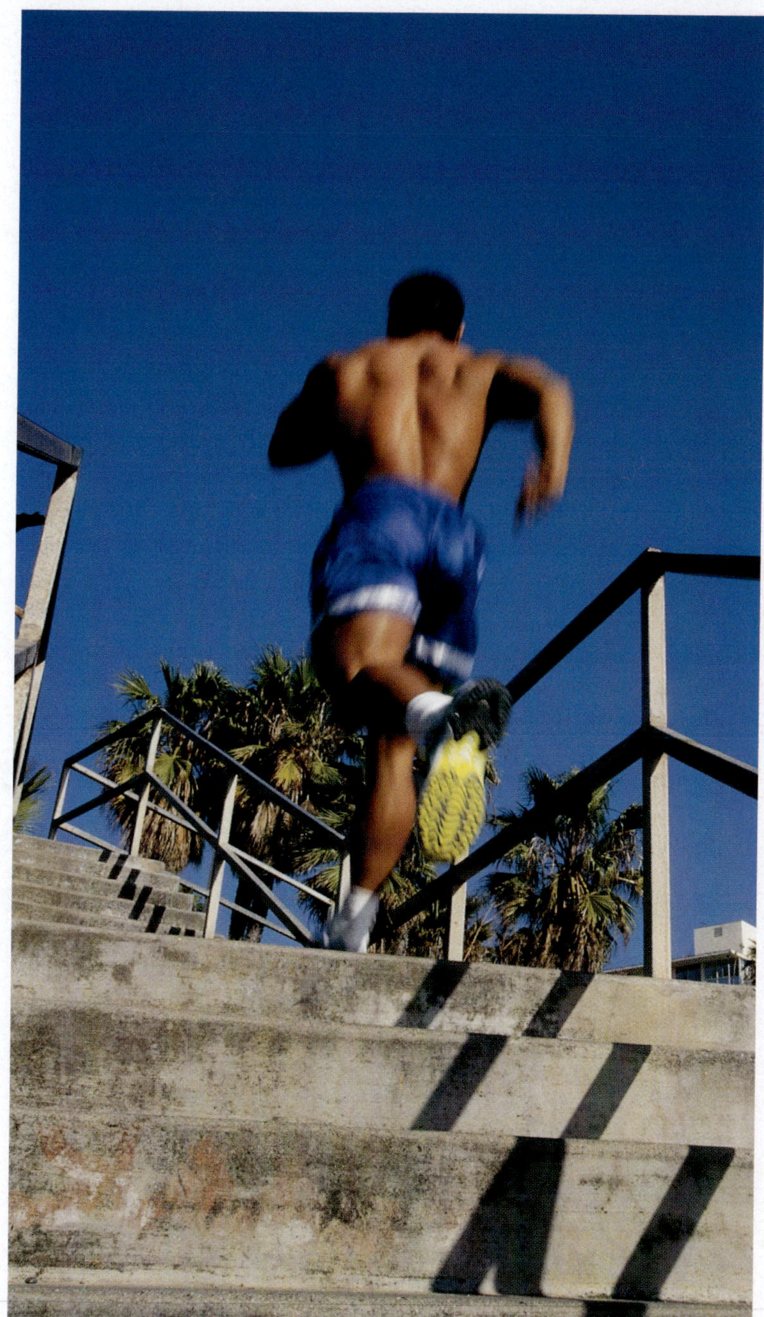

In hot weather, exercise outdoors in the morning as opposed to midday.

heat-related illnesses, including heat exhaustion, heatstroke and, in severe cases, death. It takes about 10–14 days of working or exercising in the heat for your body to adjust or become acclimatized, the American Medical Athletic Association notes, so cut down on the intensity of your exercise or activity during the first several days.

"Being 'used to' the heat or 'acclimatized' is necessary for the body to perform in hot, humid conditions without overheating," states Noel D. Nequin, MD, former president of the AMAA. "But acclimatization increases your need for fluid to match the increase in

17–20 ounces of fluid before beginning activity, and another 7–10 ounces every 10–20 minutes during activity. Consume 24 ounces of fluid within the first two hours after outdoor activity, as well. One adult-size gulp roughly equals one ounce of fluid.

To help the acclimatization process along, wear light-colored and loose-fitting clothing, and make sure you drink enough noncaffeinated and nonalcoholic fluid. Be alert for signs of severe heat illness — dry lips and tongue; headache; weakness, dizziness or extreme fatigue; concentrated urine that appears darker than normal; nausea; or muscle cramps — in yourself or

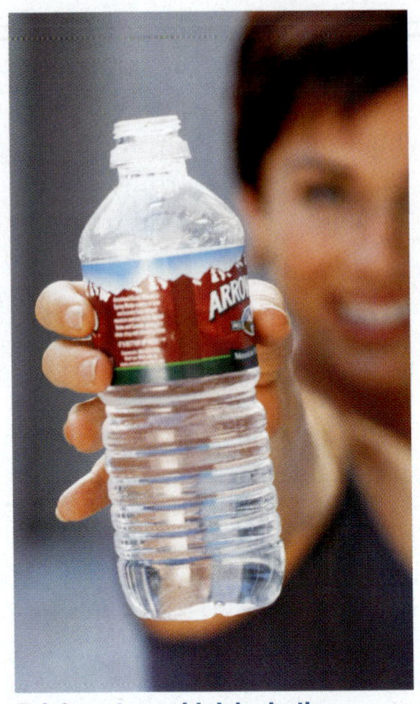

Drink up to avoid dehydration.

cooler parts of the day, like morning or evening. If you

'Be alert for signs of severe heat illness — dry lips and tongue; headache; weakness, dizziness or extreme fatigue; nausea; or muscle cramps.'

sweat rate, which puts you at higher risk for dehydration and heat illness." Adults need

another person, and seek medical attention immediately.

Also, try exercising in the

must train midday, make it indoors in an air-conditioned gym. ∎

References

1. McArdle, W., Katch, F.I., Katch, V.L. Exercise physiology: energy, nutrition and human performance. Malvern, PA: Lea & Febiger, 1991.

2. Peterson, M.S. Eat to compete. St. Louis, MO: Mosby–Year Book, 1996.

3. American College of Sports medicine position stand: The recommended quantity and quality of exercise for developing and maintaining cardiorespiratory and muscular fitness, and flexibility in healthy adults. Medicine & Science in Sports & Exercise 30(6): 975-991, 1998.

4. U.S. Department of Health and human Services. Physical activity and health: a report of the surgeon general. Atlanta, GA: U.S. Department of Health and Human Services, Centers for Disease Control and Prevention, National Center for Chronic Disease Prevention and Health Promotion, 1996.

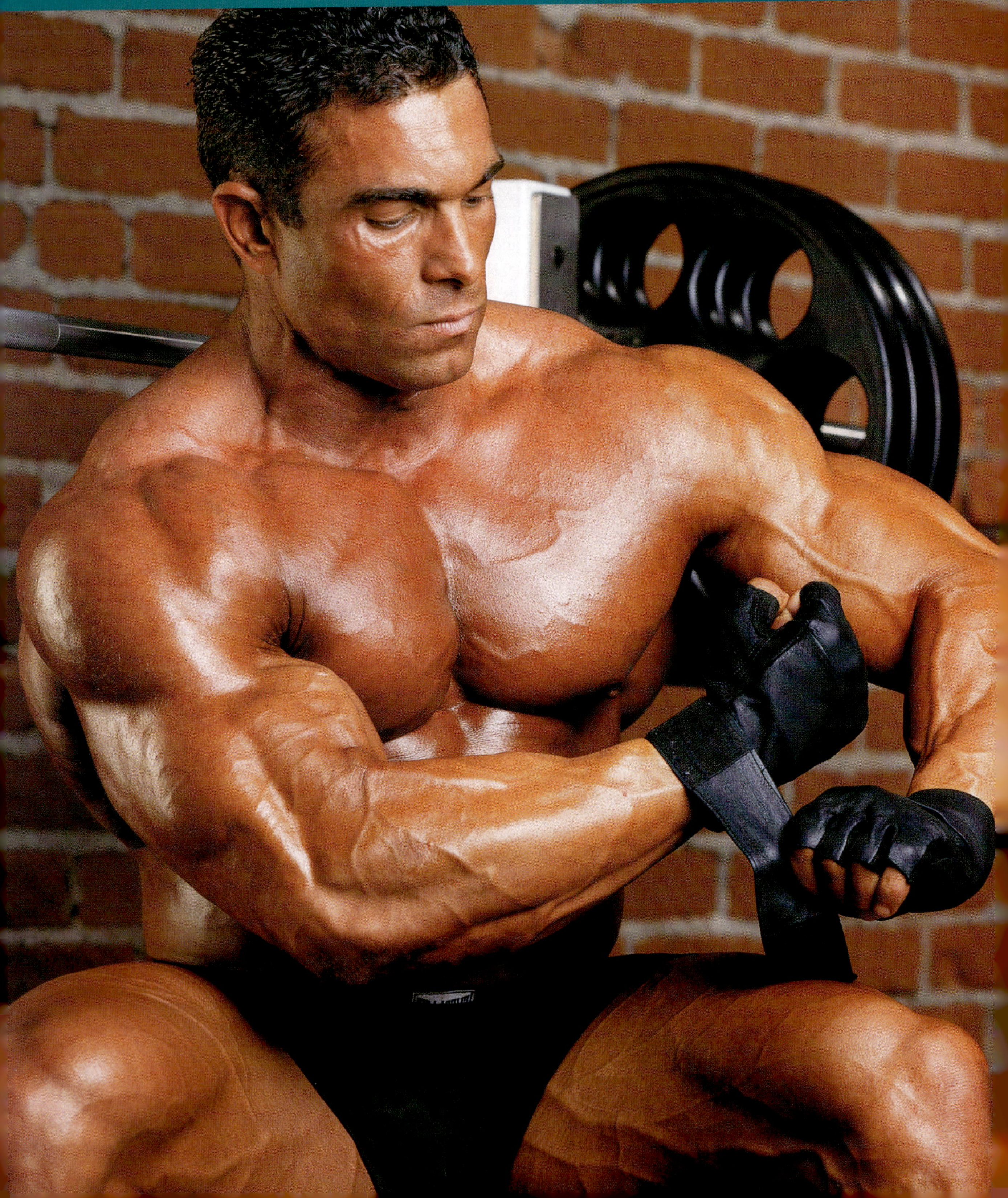

TOOLS OF THE TRADE

The essential gear from gloves to belts

In gyms and health clubs across America, you can witness a vast array of workout equipment and apparel in action. From toned trainers sporting trendy tracksuits to bulging bodybuilders wearing workout gloves and weight belts; from step instructors in halter tops and hot pants to grizzled powerlifters using hand straps and knee wraps, it seems everybody's got gear to enhance form, function or both. Which is part of why selecting the accessories that best support your workout style and goals can sometimes be a bit overwhelming. There are so many products available — some you need, some you don't — that it can be tough to find stuff that feels good, does what it's supposed to and, if you're lucky, looks cool, too.

Fortunately for you, we've dedicated this section of the book to helping you learn not only which pieces of equipment you need to build maximum muscle with minimum risk of injury, but also which products you're better off leaving on the shelf. This section covers a variety of frequently asked questions about workout accessories, such as: When should I wear a weight belt? Should I use lifting straps? Is it wise to wear knee wraps when doing heavy squats? And notwithstanding your resistance-training experience, some of the answers just

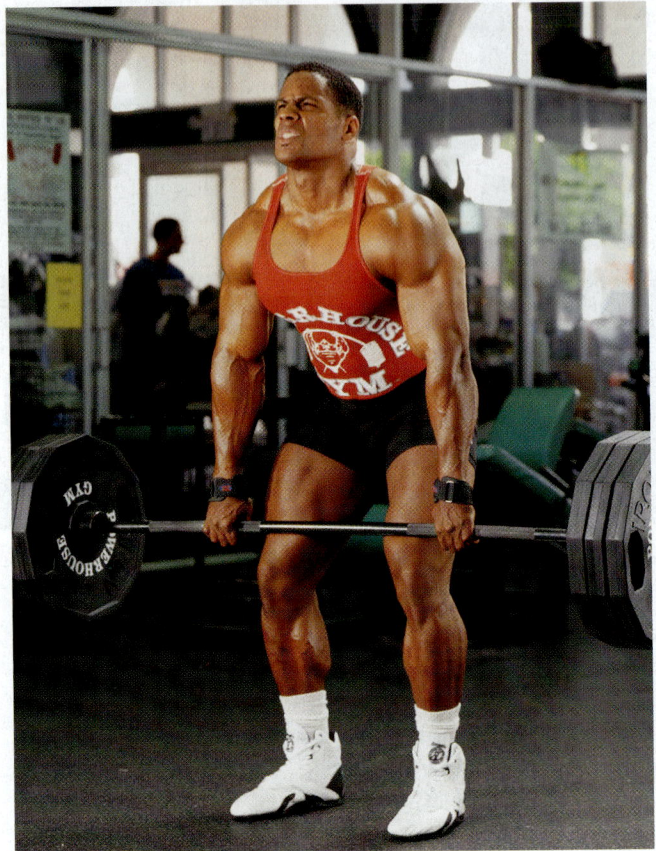

might shock you a bit. For example, did you know that using a weight belt too often could actually encourage the development of a weak midsection? Or that using straps incorrectly can get in the way of growth and reduce your forearm strength?

By addressing these sorts of questions, we'll ensure that you step into the gym with the gear you need — and the understanding of how to use it — to be successful in achieving your training goals. Additionally, we hope to provide the knowledge you must have to avoid purchasing equipment that won't benefit you in your workouts and may in fact lead to negative results and injury. After all, it's bad enough getting ripped off on an unnecessary prod-

uct; having it cause problems for you in the gym only doubles the pain.

Just so you know exactly what you're getting into, we've also provided, below, a glossary of workout equipment terms — all of which are covered in more detail in the questions and answers. If you're an intermediate or advanced lifter, you're probably already familiar with these items and can probably skip ahead. However, if you want a quick review, or if you're just getting started in weight training, these definitions will be helpful. Either way, there's little doubt that the one-minute lessons that follow will provide you with some uncommon information about resistance-training accessories, and how to use them to achieve maximum gains.

Gloves

Hand garments, often made chiefly of leather, with a Velcro strap and the fingers cut off. Used to protect the hands from developing calluses, to prevent slipping by providing a better grip on bars and other equipment, and to enhance comfort during weightlifting exercises.

Lifting straps

Heavy-duty cloth bands, usually around 1 or 1 1/2 inches across and 12 or so inches long, with a loop on one end, allowing a lifter to make a slipknot around the wrist and then wrap the remainder of the strap around a bar. Used to help a lifter hold onto barbells and dumbbells during heavy-lifting exercises such as deadlifts and rows.

Knee wraps

Heavyweight fabric strips, generally between 70 and 80 inches in length, that a lifter wraps around the knee joints. Used, often by powerlifters, to provide knee support during squats and deadlifts.

Weight-training belt

Thick leather belt, usually 4 inches wide in the back and 2 inches wide in the front. Newer belts made of softer, more flexible materials are often narrower in the back, while some powerlifters use belts that are 4 inches wide all the way around. Used to support the lower back while lifting heavy with exercises such as squats, military presses, deadlifts and bent-over rows.

Tools of the Trade: Questions and Answers

66

THE WEIGHT BELT

Should I wear a lifting belt all the time when I'm in the gym, or just during certain exercises?

A: Go into a gym almost anywhere and you'll see some hardcore bodybuilders who choose to wear belts, and others who don't. Many who are new to weight training think they need to buy belts but have no idea how they are supposed to work. Some hate to take them off. So what's the rule? After all, aside from building mass, injury-free training is a top priority for bodybuilders.

The weight belt increases intra-abdominal pressure by compressing the midsection. Increased pressure provides greater stability for the spine and discs of the lower back. Spinal stability translates into a reduced risk of injury, even when heavy weights are involved. With that said, it sounds like a weight belt should be worn at all times. Unfortunately, things aren't that simple.

Much like a weight belt, the abdominal muscles and, to a lesser degree, the muscles of the low back form a natural belt around your midsection. When contracted, these muscles squeeze the lower torso, thereby increasing intra-abdominal pressure and spinal stability. A well-conditioned midsection all but eliminates the need for a weight belt, except during lifts of maximal weight and ones that involve compressive spinal loading (such as the squat).

Here's the catch. If you use a weight belt all the time, your body

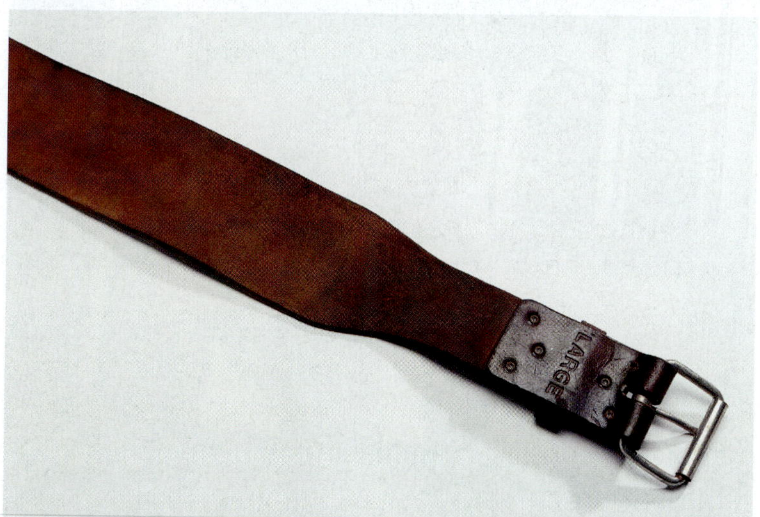

A weight belt can increase stability for the lower back during heavy lifting.

learns to rely on the belt instead of your muscles for spinal stabilization during exertion. Research has shown that the forces exerted by the muscles of the midsection decrease as the pressure applied by a belt increases.[1] With weight-belt overuse, your abdominal muscles may not be properly conditioned to provide adequate support the next time you need it (but aren't wearing a belt). The end result? Increased risk of possible low-back injury.

If you have a bad back or weak abdominal muscles, get your doctor's clearance before lifting. A weight belt may help while you're attempting overhead movements or those that require you to stand, but you should also work on strengthening your midsection with regular abdominal and low-back training. As your torso becomes stronger, use your weight belt to a lesser extent. Once you've developed a strong midsection, you'll have a permanent weight belt — made of muscle. Reserve the real weight belt for overhead lifts or any other movement that puts a heavy load on your spine (squats, deadlifts, etc.).

The use of a weight belt will be dictated by the strength of your midsection, exercise selection and the amount of weight used, but with proper training, all bodybuilders can greatly limit their need for weight belts.

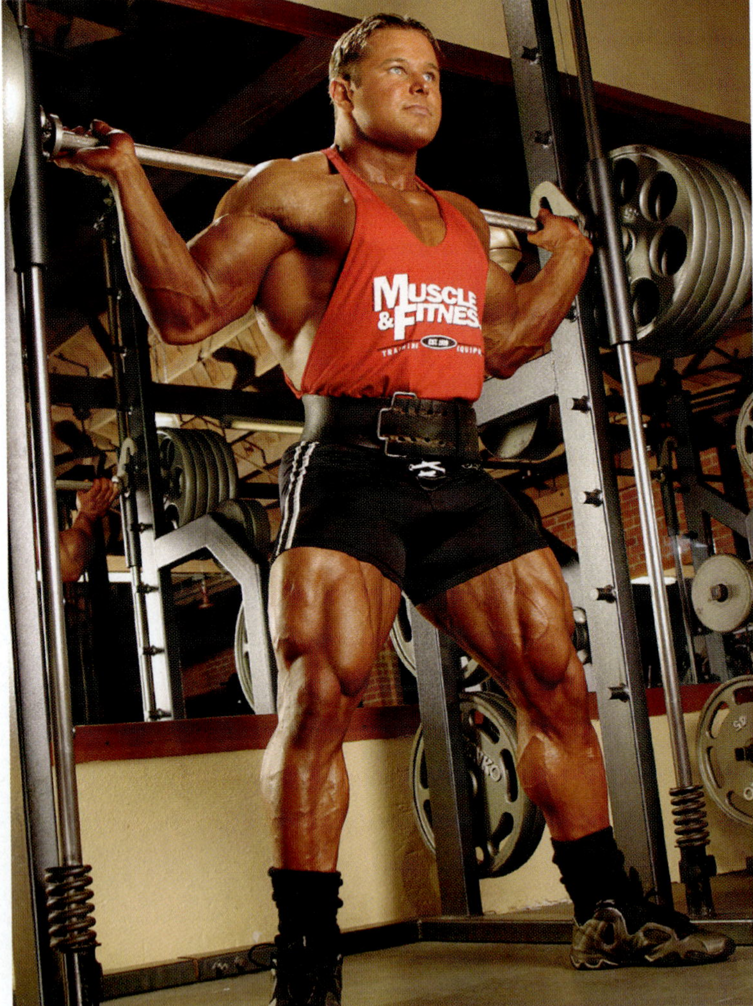

Only use a weight belt when doing moves that put great stress on your spine.

67

IT'S A WRAP

One of my knees is weaker than the other because of an operation. Is it wise to

wear knee wraps when I do heavier squats, or might it end up hurting my knee in the long run?

A: The use of knee wraps has been popularized by powerlifters squatting tons of weight; the rationale for using wraps is that they'll protect your knees from injury. Though squatting was believed to be bad for your knees many years ago, subsequent research has proven squatting to actually be good for your knees. Of course, by wrapping your knees tightly you'll end up able to squat more weight, which might be some people's primary reason for using them.

Your concerns may be different. If your knee problem was centered around a common area — anterior/posterior cruciate ligament, meniscus or tendon — you should be mainly concerned with strengthening your weaker knee to a degree where it matches the strength of your healthy knee.

Says William Post, MD, assistant professor and chief of sports medicine and shoulder surgery in the department of orthopedics at West Virginia University School of Medicine in Morgantown, "For patients and athletes to return to their desired activity level, their rehabilitated strength and flexibility must often exceed the preinjury level, since that level was inadequate to support the original loads imposed." What this basically means is that you need to pump iron with the goal of getting bigger and stronger. But Post goes on to say, "The cocontractions [of all muscles involved] and weight-bearing loads associated with closed-chain activities [such as squatting] tend to be tolerated better than open-chain exercise [like leg extensions] in most patients with patellofemoral disorders." [2]

So, now that you know you should indeed train and can also squat, how do you best go about it? This may come as a surprise: Using knee wraps is probably counterproductive in your case, particularly if you wrap only the previously injured knee. What you end up doing is providing artificial support to the knee, robbing its supportive structures of the stimulus needed to grow stronger.

Richard T. Herrick, MD, an orthopedic surgeon and actively competing masters weightlifter and powerlifter, explains: "The use of wraps isn't even needed in instances of knee rehabilitation. However, if you feel the need to increase warmth to the area, using a knee sleeve can be a good thing to do. If you feel there's a significant degree of strength imbalance between the knees, you need to pay particular attention to not shifting the emphasis to the stronger leg. If you can, work through the entire range of motion; if not, just go as deep as you can pain-free and slowly work your way down to a full squat over time."

Herrick advises starting with a weight with which you can do three sets of 10 reps, then increasing it. Once you can com-

'Knee wraps end up providing artificial support to the knee, robbing its supportive structures of the stimulus needed to grow stronger.'

plete another three sets of 10, increase the weight again. After the imbalance subsides, you can slowly begin to hit the weights even harder.

A lot of knee injuries can be traced back to overwork. In our zeal to get as big and strong as possible, we often overlook the value of rest. When that happens, our bodies aren't able to recuperate to the degree necessary for subsequent training sessions. An added dilemma is that when your body gets tired, technique tends to falter. This is the perfect prescription for injury. To avoid it, be sure you allow for sufficient rest between workouts — at least three days before hitting the same bodypart again.

Also consider lowering the volume and intensity of your work periodically to allow sufficient rest, and think technique, technique, technique. You should also incorporate various stretches into your program. By ensuring that your quads and hamstrings are flexible and able to functionally work through the full range of motion, you'll give your knees additional tools for getting stronger and more balanced. And talking about hamstrings, training them is very important because they play a vital role in balancing your thigh strength and preventing injury.

Bottom line, knee wraps aren't needed to strengthen your knee and can actually be counterproductive. Save the knee wraps for when your knee is completely healed and as strong as the other one and you decide to push some very heavy weights.

68

STRAPPED FOR DEVELOPMENT

I've been using lifting straps for quite some time; they help me hold onto the bar and I can get a couple of more reps that way. I mostly use them on pull-downs, chins and rows, and sometimes on barbell curls when I go heavy. But it just occurred to me that I could be weakening my grip. What do you think?

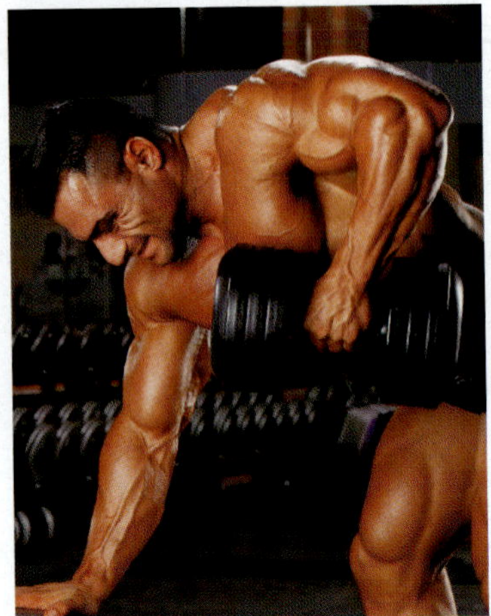
To develop your grip strength, lift heavy weights without straps.

A: Definitely. Barring any type of injury, why would anyone want to use anything that would on one hand make them lift more and on the other create a weakness. Bodybuilding is about developing strength and size in all areas. Lifting straps don't allow for this.

As you can probably imagine, grip strength is essential in many exercises as well as in any manual labor you might do. To develop your grip, simply train without straps. Sure, in the beginning you may not get as many reps as before, but just look at it as needed recuperation time. Before too long, you'll be able to hold onto the bar regardless of weight and number of reps.

One limiting factor may be the bar. You see, if you do pull-downs, you probably use a fixed bar that doesn't rotate. Yet in certain exercises that require a regular barbell, such as rows, the bar will tend to roll out of your hands when you use an overhand grip. This may happen with a dumbbell, too, and certainly presents a challenge. I'd go as heavy and do as many reps as possible without straps, then use straps for maybe your last 1–2 sets. Be sure, however, to decrease your use of straps over time. Once you're able to hold onto the bar until the main muscle group you're exercising is fatigued, you'll know you've developed a vise-like grip.

You can also specifically train your grip by going beyond wrist curls and hammer curls. Pinch-grip two 25-pound plates, buy yourself some heavy-duty grippers, or even use a wire cutter at home to cut through thick wire several times — you'll get quite a pump. In addition, you could set a barbell in the power rack at about knee height and simply lift it with one hand off the pins for a 15-count. Once you can do a 25-count, move up in weight.

69

GET A GRIP

Do gloves make much of a difference in your grip? Some of the guys use them at my gym, but I think it's because they want to look hardcore.

A: A chain is only as strong as its weakest link. And when it comes to training, the body works as a chain in a series of links. One weak point throws the whole system off.

In any exercise performed correctly, the working muscles are assisted by everything from your abs to your lower back to your posture to your grip. If anything in that whole-body equa-

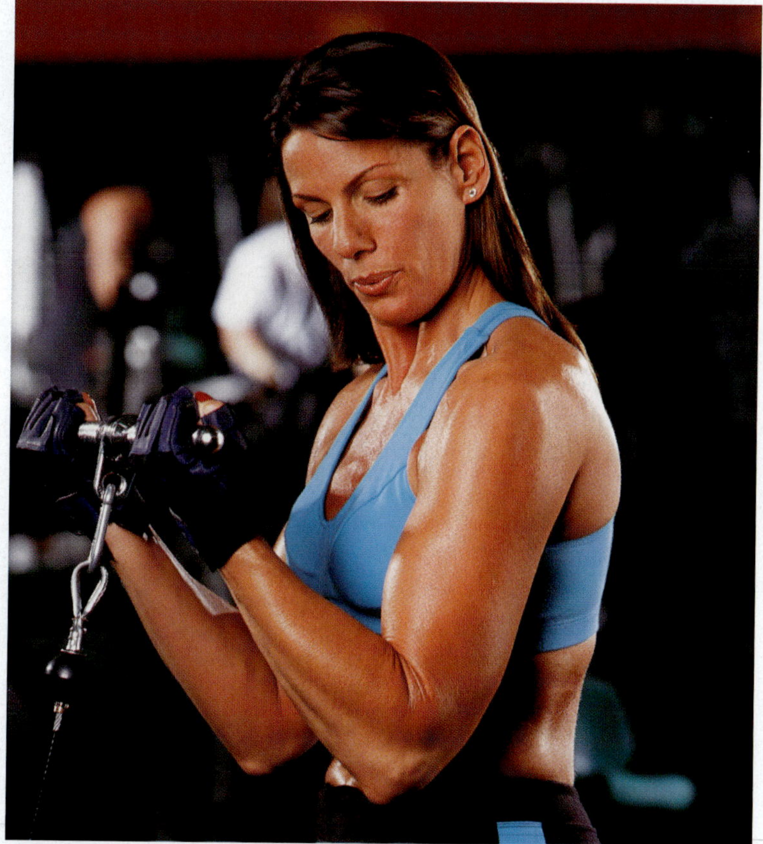

Gloves can enhance your grip and help prevent the development of calluses.

tion is weaker than the muscles you're targeting, guess what? Your failing grip will make you kiss your set goodbye. Thankfully, a few choice accessories can enable you to vote off your weak spots so you emerge stronger, bigger and better.

Get a Grip

Gloves are a simple way to solve a variety of problems at the gym that would otherwise put a crimp in your training, particularly for exercises such as curls and pulls. "In many cases, gloves enable exercisers to maintain a better grip on the bar, especially if their hands are sweaty," notes fitness competitor and personal trainer Laura Mak, MS, CSCS. The last thing you want to worry about is grip slippage due to sweat; wearing gloves can keep your mind on the lift rather than on your sweaty palms. Preventing calluses is another primary reason to wear gloves during a workout.

The Bottom Line

• Choose a leather glove with high-quality stitching.

• Most gloves can be handwashed in warm water with a few drops of mild detergent; air dry on a flat surface.

• If sweat is a concern, look for gloves with moisture-wicking technology.

70

FIT TO BE TRAINED

What do you recommend for comfort and performance in gym wear? I'm kind of overweight, so there's no way I'm going to be wearing any skin-tight fashions, but some sweatsuits are too heavy and I get too hot. Any ideas?

A: A few factors are important when deciding what to wear during your workouts. First, do your clothes match

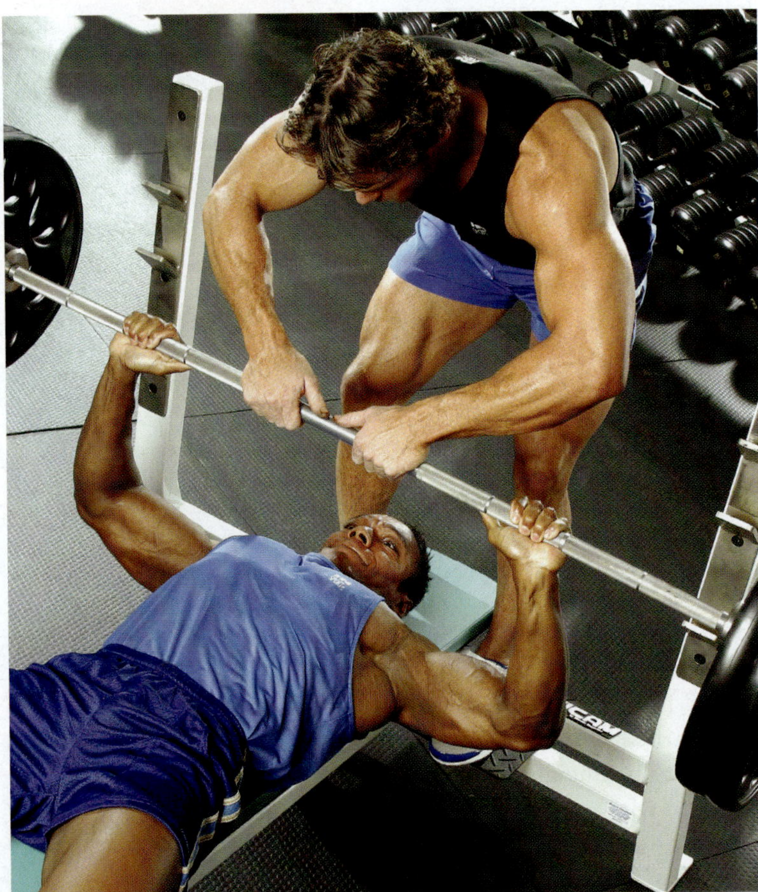

Good workout clothes are comfortable, safe and made of breathable fabrics.

the temperature of your training area? Scientists tell us that a slightly warm gym is best for training because it's good for blood circulation (and therefore between-set recovery) and you will get a better training effect when the temperature is on the warm side. So choose your clothes to fit this temperature suggestion. If your gym is cool, wear a sweatsuit, and if it's hot, dress down to a T-shirt and shorts. Fabric can make a big difference in you level of comfort.

Look for workout clothes made out of cotton and breathable synthetics, which work best because they cool and either absorb or wick away perspiration.

Next, your clothes should be comfortable and safe. Wearing clothes that are too loose may hinder training technique by binding up during full range movements and get caught on obstacles in your gym area. And wearing clothes that are too tight or restrictive may hinder training technique and restrict blood flow. So make sure your clothing is loose enough or elastic enough to allow you to stretch thoroughly.

Last, don't underestimate the importance of what's on your feet. Your shoes must be supportive when under heavy iron. They should have solid arch supports, and not easily flex laterally or "roll" to the sides while lifting. This is not only dangerous because you may get hurt, it can also cause chronic knee, hip and ankle problems. ■

References

1. Lander, J.E, Simonton, R.L, Giacobbe, J.K. The effectiveness of weight belts during the squat exercise. Medicine & Science in Sports & Exercise 22(1): 117-126, 1990.

2. Post, W.R. Patellofemoral pain: let the physical exam define treatment. The Physician and Sportsmedicine 26(1): 68-78, 1998.

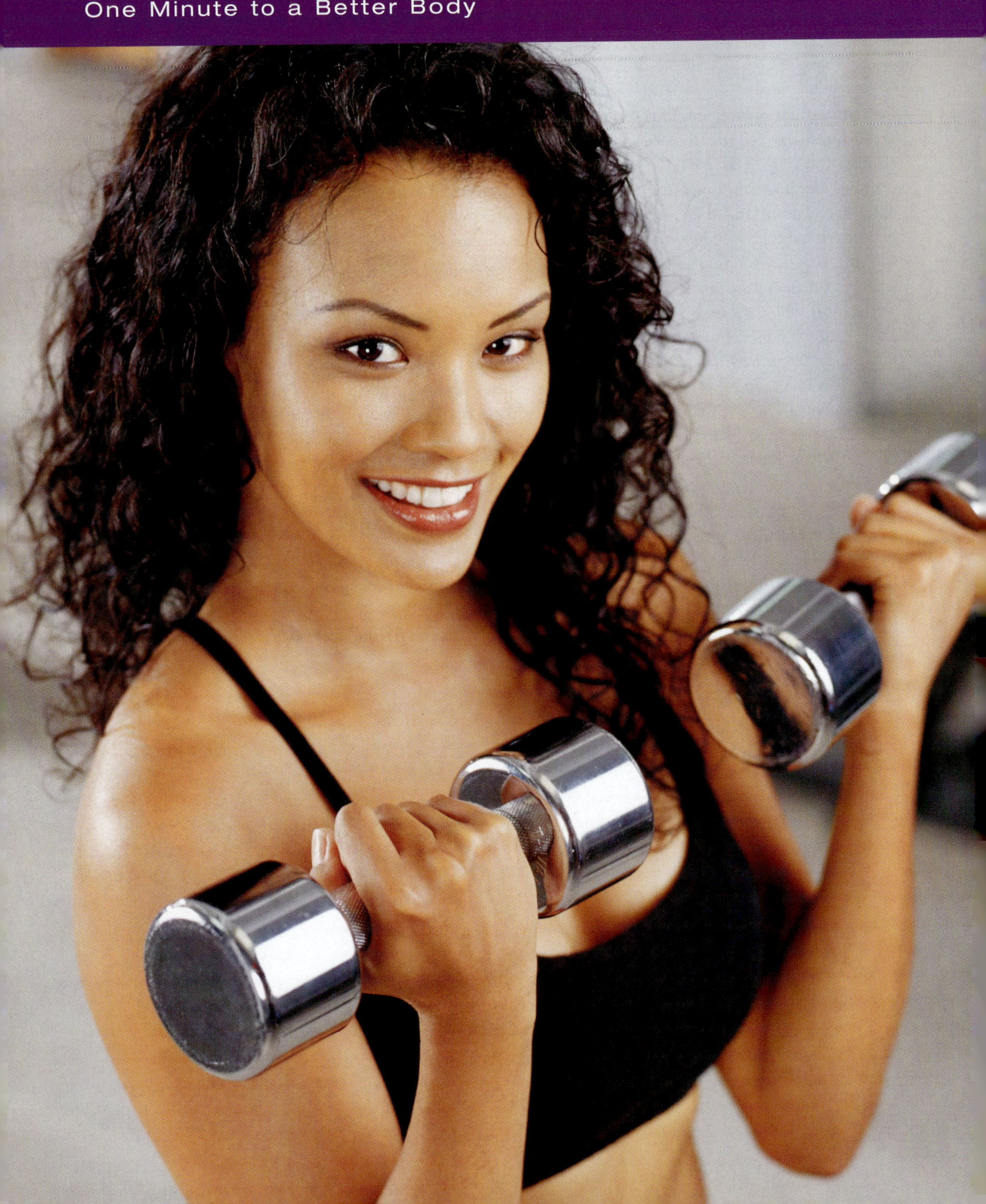

WOMEN IN THE WEIGHT ROOM

Fine-tuned training tips for her

A number of head-to-toe differences make it important for men and women to train differently. In fact, knowing your body gives you clues about how to build muscle in the right areas while you avoid adding fat in the wrong ones. Here's a top-down approach to the differences in metabolism between men and women and how they affect you as an athlete.

Head

Where fat is concerned, scientists say it's all in your head. Apparently, a chorus line of hormones acting in the brain regulate bodyfat in both men and women. The most famous of these is leptin, and women have more of it than men in part because they have more fat (fat cells make leptin to speed fat breakdown).[1] Indeed, this may be part of the reason women tend to use more fat as a fuel source during exercise while men favor carbs.[2]

Other than leptin, many anabolic hormones and hormones that cause the release of anabolic hormones originate in the brain. For example, growth

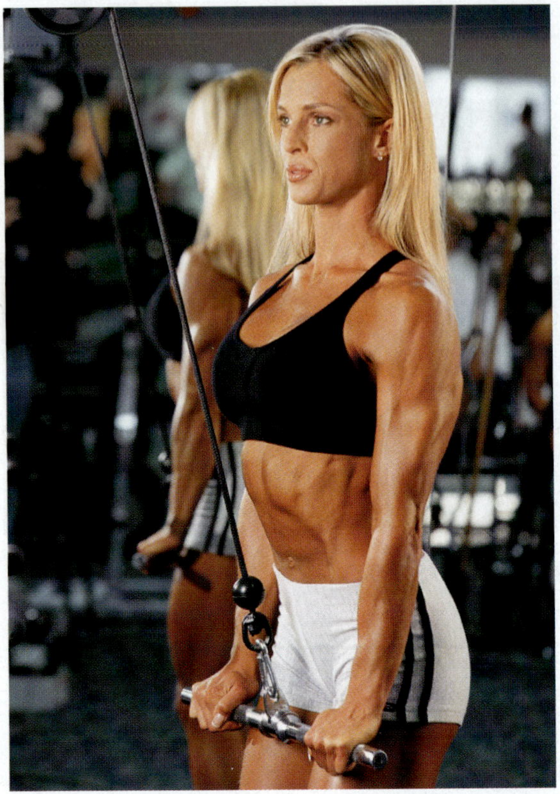

Muscle

Women tend to have less muscle and more fat than men, and as a result they have less space in which to store muscle carbs (glycogen) and more space in which to store fat. (Women also have 20% smaller livers than men; the liver is a key organ for glycogen storage.)

In addition, women protect their glycogen stores more than men. One spin-off is that women may benefit less from carb loading before a sports event than men. For example, eating 75% of calories from carbs vs. 60% for four days before a triathlon bolstered glycogen levels in men (by 41%) but not in women.[3]

Even so, women and men are more similar than different where bodybuilding is concerned. Changes in muscle structure are fairly consistent in both males and females following weight training.[4] Women may or may not have a greater proportion of fat-burning slow-twitch muscle fibers than men, but because women have less muscle, their energy needs are about 10% less relative to their weight and they don't need to eat as many calories as men.

Blood

Women have more trouble than men generating as much calorie-burning intensity while exercising, even when their smaller body size is taken into account. This is partly because women's muscles aren't as well supplied with oxygen-rich blood. Women have fewer small blood vessels (capillaries) nourishing each muscle, and their blood is less rich in oxygen-carrying hemoglobin.[5] Nonetheless, women have a variety of ways to make up for this in their training.

Adrenal Glands

Men burn more calories at rest than women because they have more muscle. Yet that isn't the whole picture; men also release more of the fat-burning hormones adrenalin and noradrenaline

hormone is released from the pituitary gland (found in the brain), and luteinizing hormone from the same area causes the release of testosterone from the testes. Testosterone's effect on brain aggression levels might explain why men have less trouble pushing themselves to peak intensity during a workout than women.

Interestingly, women partially make up for lower testosterone levels by having much higher growth hormone (GH) levels. But while men's GH levels rise when they exercise, women's GH levels don't. For this and other reasons, women should combine exercise with a diet of whole foods, portion control and dietary restraint for successful weight loss. In regard to exercise, women may benefit greatly from circuit and interval training.

(aka norepinephrine, the hormone increased by taking ephedrine). The thermogenic effect of norepinephrine is one reason men burn "hotter" than women.[6] Along the same lines, men's bodies give a better adrenalin pump with train-

fat, it's important to set realistic standards.

Men usually have less fat overall than women, and carry a greater proportion of it in and on their upper body (in visceral and abdominal fat stores). This is believed to be due to a high ratio

'Because women's bodies don't release as many fat-burning hormones in response to exercise, they must be stricter with their diets.'

ing. The result is a greater rise in blood pressure and an increased fat-burning boost.[7]

Because women's bodies don't release as many fat-burning hormones in response to exercise, they must be stricter with their diets. Men, on the other hand, get more bang from their buck with exercise where fat loss is concerned. Happily, women can compensate by pushing themselves harder, at which point they can release as much noradrenaline as men do.[8] Adding interval training is one way to do this; short bursts of high-intensity exercise cause noradrenaline release, which leads to a loss of up to 100 extra calories as heat in the hours following exercise.

Fat

Men and women need to be judged differently where fat is concerned, since 7%–8% of a woman's bodyfat involves breast tissue and reproductive stores needed to support healthy ovulation each month. Since another 4% is essential fat needed to pad vital organs, no woman should go below about 11% bodyfat for any reason. A man, however, can go as low as 4% for short periods. In one study, the average female bodybuilder was found to have 13.2% bodyfat, while male bodybuilders averaged 9.3%. Since most women look slim at 17% body-

of testosterone to estrogen.

Most women store fat on their hips, thighs and buttocks as well as their breasts, similarly due to sex hormone differences.[9] Yet loss of thigh fat in women may be further complicated by an excess of alpha-2 receptors relative to men. These alpha-2 receptors switch off the release of fat-burning noradrenaline, and are believed to make it tough

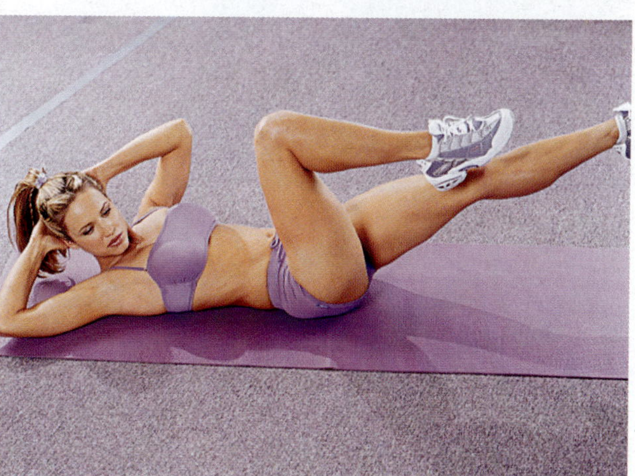

for women to lose thigh fat even when other areas of their bodies may slim down. Intense, muscle-sparing resistance exercise combined with a supplement called yohimbine may help, but yohimbine shouldn't be used in conjunction with ephedrine and caffeine. While it blocks alpha-2 receptors (at least in a test tube) and has been recommended for loss of fat from the thighs, this use is unproven: Yohimbine hasn't been tested on living women nor shown to reduce thigh fat.

Sex Organs

In both sexes, testosterone levels increase with intense bodybuilding training, although grueling, long-term cardio reduces testosterone lev-

testosterone-trapping protein sex-hormone-binding globulin (SHBG), which increases with training. This further reduces free testosterone, but women somewhat compensate for their low levels of anabolic testosterone by having higher GH levels. Interestingly, men have a more robust GH response to exercise than women.[10]

Metabolism

One advantage women enjoy over men is

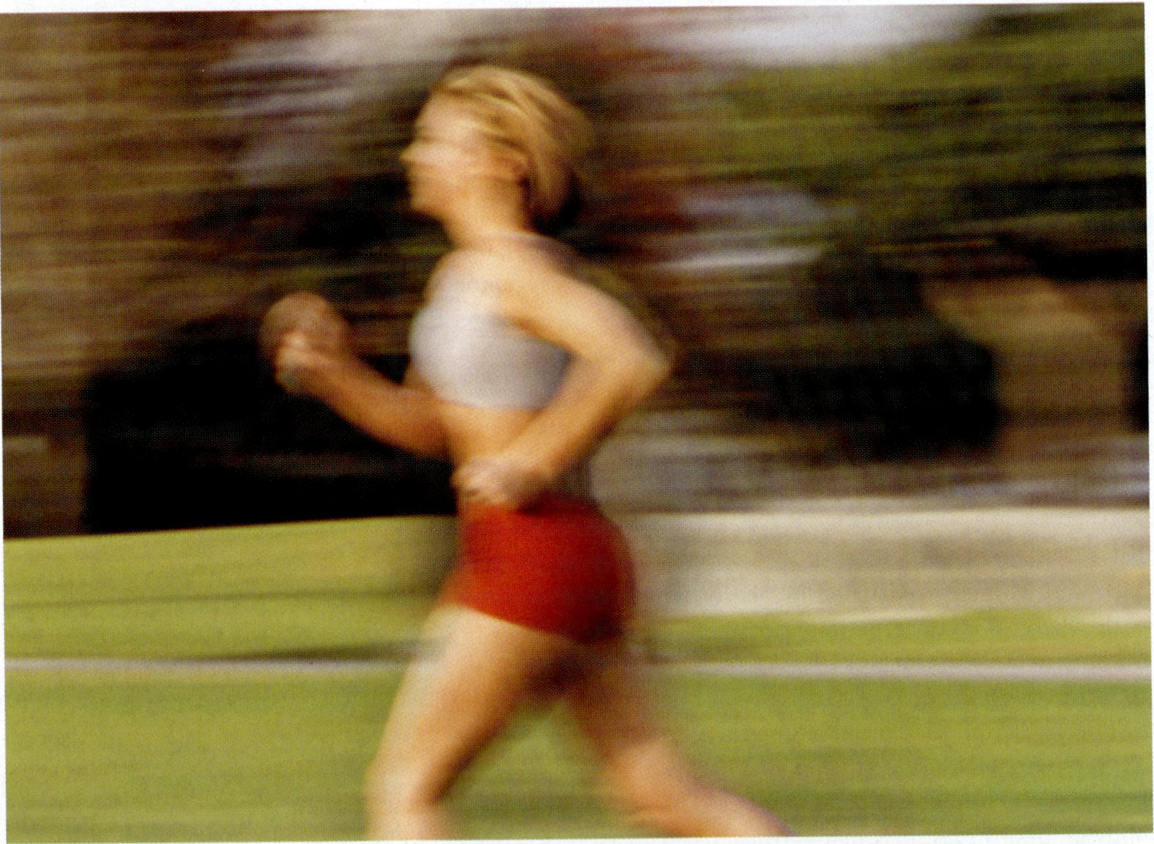

els. Men show a greater testosterone rise in response to intense exercise than women and have 10 times as much to begin with. Furthermore, women have higher levels of the

monthly surges in progesterone during the luteal phase before menstruation. Apparently, progesterone is thermogenic, and a significant number of extra calories are burned by women at this time of the month when body temperature goes up. This explains why women may be able to get away with eating an extra 300 calories per day before menstruation (providing ovulation actually occurs).[11]

Genes

Besides the obvious difference between men and women at their 23rd pair of chromosomes known as the sex chromosomes (women have XX and men have XY), genes in their muscle cells also differ. A study out of the University of Pittsburgh discovered that men have higher expression of more than 175 genes in their muscles as compared to women. The majority of these genes produce proteins that are involved in the structural and metabolic components of the muscle cell. Typically, the higher the expression of the gene, the greater the amount of the protein produced for that particular function (whether it's contraction or metabolism). Stephen Roth, PhD, postdoctoral fellow in the department of human genetics, and lead author on the study published in the journal Physiological Genomics, adds: "Very little work has been done to characterize molecular differences between men and women for skeletal muscle tissue, and our findings are some of the first to suggest that significant differences do exist. Future work will need to focus on specific genes with known gender differences in expression, with the idea that such differences could potentially explain differences in the response of muscle to exercise observed between men and women." Someday women may be able to turn on the genes that limit their growth potential, eliminating the term "the weaker sex."

Women in the Weight Room: Questions and Answers

TONE, NOT BULK

I want to get toned, but not big and bulky. Should I avoid weights so I won't end up looking like a man?

A: Women, listen up. If you take one vitally important beauty tip into the world after reading this, it should be that a little muscle is a good thing. Trust us. Not only does it keep you looking youthful and sexy but, more important, it makes you feel youthful, sexy, strong and confident. Muscle also burns more calories, prevents skin from sagging and maintains youthful contours and curves.

Darn thing is, ask any personal trainer what the most commonly heard remark is from a woman about to embark upon her initial journey into the world of weights: "I don't want to get too big." Fat chance. Most women don't have enough

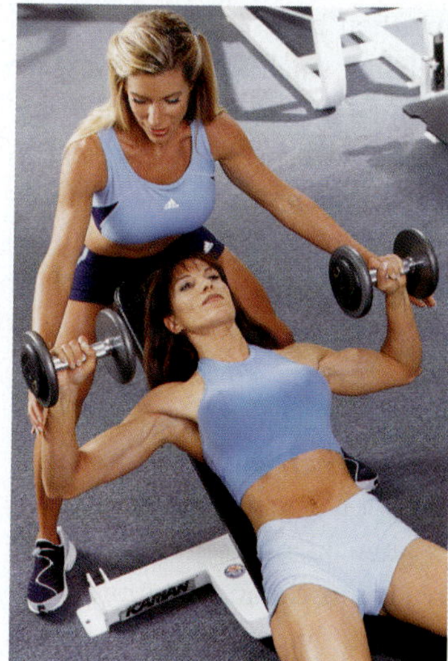
Building muscle with weight training will help you burn more calories.

testosterone to grow huge naturally, and it takes great effort — superclean eating and superintense training, consistently and over an extended period — to just build some feminine-looking mass.

Ironically, the "toned" look that fills our dreams is nothing but muscle in all its beauty. So, please, stop fretting about miraculously morphing into a 170-pound pro bodybuilder with (gasp!) pecs puffed out like the hills of Kentucky. Won't happen.

Lifting heavy will not make you look like a bodybuilder! In fact, the majority of women who aren't progressing aren't lifting enough weight. They're so afraid of bulking up that they stick to those 3- and 5-pound weights and are actually impeding their progress.

Using small weights for a few months when you're first starting out is fine, but after that, you're not challenging your muscles any more and are pretty much wasting your time. Progress slowly to heavier weights so your muscles are continually challenged. You won't get big, but you will get denser and stronger, and you'll get "toned," as most women like to call it. "Tone" is really muscle, and the more muscle you have, the better you'll look and the faster your metabolic rate will be.

72

DIFFERENT STROKES FOR FEMALE FOLKS

I was doing deadlifts at the gym the other day when a guy came up to me and said that that wasn't a good exercise for women. Is he right? Are there specific exercises for women?

A: You've hit on a popular issue. Considering that our muscles' characteristics aren't different from a man's for the most part, and that several training studies show similar muscle growth patterns between the genders, there is no evidence suggesting we should train any differently than men. So if you're trying to build an effective routine, look at what the strongest and smartest guy does in the gym, make some slight adjustments to meet your personal needs and expect to make progress like never before.

When you want to personalize your routine, periodize your program by altering your exercise choice, sets, repetitions, intensity and rest. (See "Not Your Usual Routine" in section 2). Use mainly multijoint and multiplane free-weight exercises to optimize neuromuscular coordination,

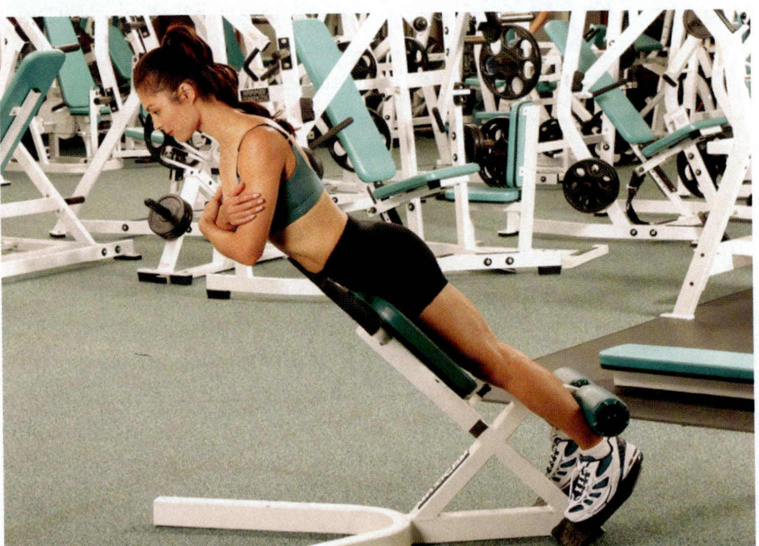

Back extensions should be a part of every woman's upper-body routine.

'Periodize your program by altering your exercise choice, sets, repetitions, intensity and rest.'

movement patterns, balance and speed. For your lower body, incorporate free-weight exercises that emphasize foot-based (closed-chain) exercises, such as lunges and squats (as opposed to leg extensions). Your upper-body exercises should include, among other things, bench and incline presses, pull-downs, pull-ups, back extensions, curls, pressdowns and abdominal work.[12] Try advanced exercises such as power cleans, hang cleans, push presses, snatches, and clean and jerks after you develop a solid strength base.

Speaking of strength, you may be interested to know that your strength gains occur basically at the same rate as for men.[13,14,15] Now, you may have heard this many times before: Women have less absolute muscle mass in their upper bodies compared to men. This is true when you eliminate bodyfat and compare strength to lean body mass. But if you were to look at a specific muscle, things might not be so clear-cut. One study trained the biceps in both genders for 20 weeks and found that the women actually showed greater relative strength increases than the men, even though muscle size increased similarly between

the genders.[16] Certainly puzzling, but evidence that you just can't make broad generalizations.

Looking at the lower body, it has been speculated but not scientifically supported that a woman's broader hips and an increased Q-angle (hip-to-knee angle) may give us an advantage in squatting exercises.[17] If you look at the lower body in terms of leg strength relative to lean body mass, some studies show we may even be stronger than men.[13]

So keep on bodybuilding to optimize what you've got, and hope that your genes support you in your quest.

73

FEMALE MOTIVATION

I'd like to join a gym and a friend suggested a women-only gym near my home. What are the benefits of a gym like this? Is it better to work out in a co-ed facility?

A: Deciding on a gym these days isn't dissimilar to buying a new car. Pushy salespeople, flashy new products and innumerable added electives all need to be factored into your decision-making process. The problem is further compounded for us women, who have yet another option to consider: co-ed or women-only.

Male Motivation & the Meet Market

While serious training and getting fit are important issues to women in both types of facilities, socializing with the opposite sex may be the greatest appeal of a co-ed gym atmosphere.

The presence or absence of the opposite sex can make or break your workout experience, depending on your personal preference. Some women find that they push themselves harder when they are around men.

Some women, however, don't feel the need for male reinforcement. So while some women are driven by men, so do men drive others away.

Members of female facilities often join to relieve negative pressures such as self-consciousness, embarrassment and intimidation that they feel in the presence of guys.

Some women find they feel like they are ogled at co-ed facilities and enjoy a women-only gym because they feel it's easier to relax and concentrate on their goals.

Weighty Issues

Although part of your decision will undoubtedly be based on the comfort level and social attitude of a club, many practical details should also be considered. Ask yourself: Does this gym offer what I want, when I want it, and how I like it? This may sound like a bad advertisement for a fast-food burger, but before dropping a hefty down-payment on a membership, reflect on these essential elements:

Crowded House: Cardio machines and hot equipment pieces in large facilities may be monopolized during peak hours. The size of a facility and the amount of available equipment are usually in direct proportion. So if you prefer a co-ed atmosphere but hate crowds, check into the larger clubs or go during off-peak times.

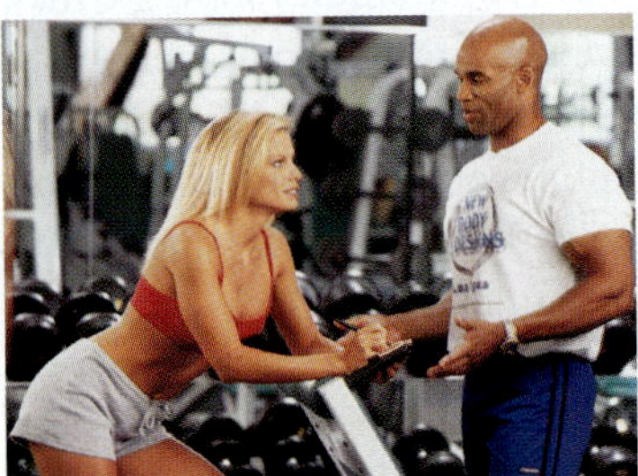

Personal trainers can be invaluable.

Pay Attention: Most gyms offer personal training services; however, all-female facilities generally don't allow male trainers on staff to maintain the comfort level of their clientele. Again, the choice is personal, and male trainers can be as invaluable and inspiring to clients as women.

Class Act: The availability and types of classes offered may be of concern to you aerobics junkies out there. While most clubs offer several class choices, all-female gyms tend to be more gender-specific with their selection. Ask for a week's pass to test-drive some of the classes offered at the gym you're considering.

Price Club: Despite the general misconception that all-women facilities are higher in cost, most have competitive pricing, comparable specials and similar deals as the co-ed gyms. The variations depend greatly on the extra amenities offered at each club, regardless of the gender trend.

Juggling Junior: If you're a mom, the availability of child care will undoubtedly affect your decision. Many gyms offer babysitting and day-care, with the women-only facilities being the more consistent of the two in terms of services available. Be sure to look into the hours and days of available care before making your gym choice, as they're sometimes limited.

Bottom Line

Whichever type you choose, your gym should meet your personality, expectations and requirements. The right facility can inspire tenacity and garner positive results. So shop around, have fun and good luck!

'Ask yourself: Does this gym offer what I want, when I want it, and how I like it?'

74

TIMING ISN'T EVERYTHING

Is it safe to lift weights when I have my period? If so, will this time of month affect my gains positively or negatively?

A: Experiencing menstruation is a clear difference between us and the guys. Not much evidence exists on how the menstrual cycle affects strength training,[18,19] though it's generally accepted that no significant negative effects should be expected.[14,20] In 1993, William J. Kraemer, PhD, CSCS, and colleagues from Pennsylvania State University found that women had higher resting growth-hormone (GH) levels during the days immediately following menstruation compared to growth-hormone levels in males.[13] This is important because GH will affect skeletal muscle growth in response to weight training,[18] but shouldn't be interpreted to mean that you'll grow more at that time of the month. Another study found that women significantly increased their quadriceps and grip strength during the mid-cycle (ovulation),[21] but more research is needed for more conclusive evidence. For now, don't let your cycle dictate what kind of day you'll have in the gym.

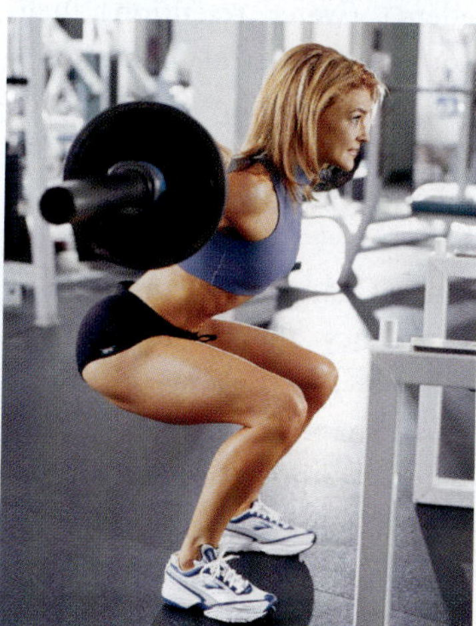

Continue strength training no matter where you are in your cycle.

75

DOUBLE TROUBLE

I've been losing weight for the past year and am almost satisfied with my shape. My only complaint is that my breasts have gotten smaller, to the point that they're almost nonexistent. I've added some fat back into my diet, but any weight I gain goes elsewhere. Short of getting implants, is there anything I can do?

A:  Bonnie Modugno, MS, RD, owner of NutritionWorks (Santa Monica, CA) offers some general observations. First, the problem could be a consequence both of being underweight and training hard. If you're chronically undereating for your body size and activity level, that could affect your breast size. Under that scenario, the fat content of your diet wouldn't be the overriding concern. Look at the number of calories you're taking in relative to how much you're training.

Genetic factors also come into play. Watching the Olympics, you will notice that virtually all the female triathletes are small-breasted. It might be a result of their intense training, or it might be self-selection: that is, a small-breasted body tends to be more ectomorphic, and an ectomorphic body is well-suited for running distances, etc. So your genetic predisposition to breast size can't be discounted.

Since you appear to have been

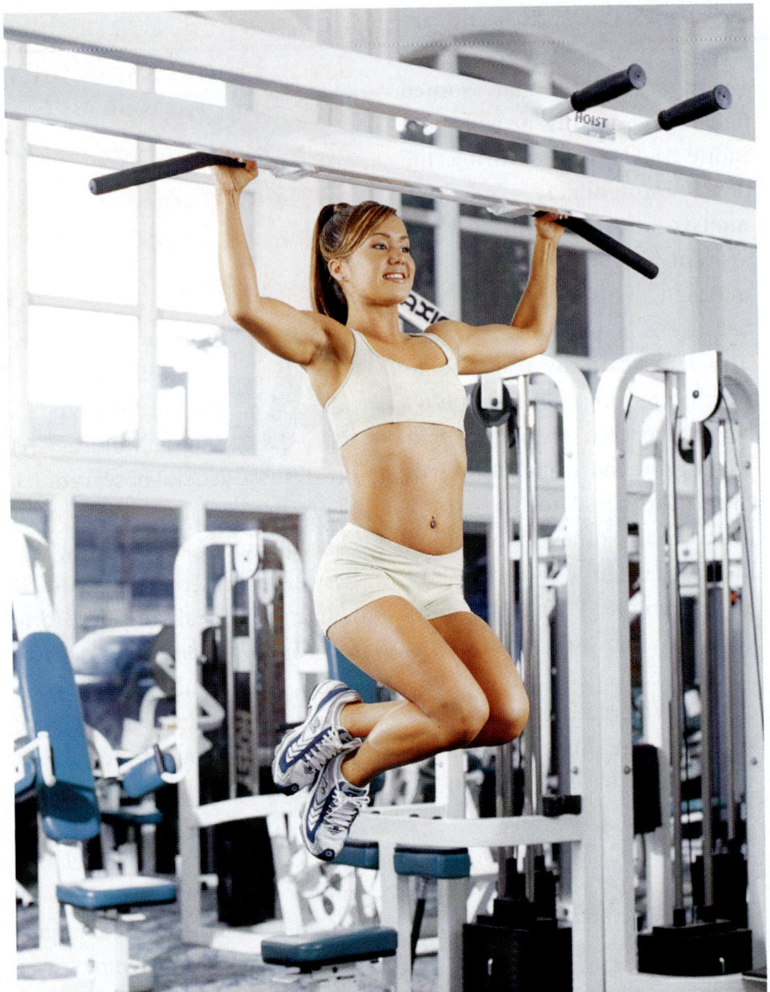

Small breasts are often a necessary trade-off of a super-lean physique.

relatively content with your breast size before you started losing weight, focus on training and diet. Training really hard and consuming insufficient calories for your activity level will definitely contribute to smaller breasts. Remember, too, that trade-offs are at work here.

If you want, say, 12% or less bodyfat as a means to achieving a chiseled six-pack, you probably can't have naturally large breasts, too. The two just don't go together. Very few women who are extremely lean still have a significant amount of breast tissue.

76

GREAT EXPECTATIONS

I'm thrilled to be pregnant, but unsure about how to alter my training routine. Is it safe to keep working out?

A: Forget about sitting it out. Pregnancy is a crucial time for fitness. Exercise during pregnancy can make you feel better and stay healthier. It helps to prevent excessive weight gain, decrease stress, relieve constipation and minimize muscle stiffness. It can reduce or prevent edema (water retention), help you sleep better at night, lessen fatigue, maintain strong back muscles and improve your mental and emotional outlook.

Many Changes Coming

Pregnancy alters your body in many ways. Besides changing your shape, it increases your blood volume, body temperature and metabolic rate, as well as resting heart rate and oxygen consumption. All of this affects your training. During exercise, blood flow may be diverted from the baby to the working muscles, and maternal body temperature and metabolic rate may rise too much. Problems such as hypoxia (low oxygen levels), hyperthermia (high body temperature), hypoglycemia (low blood sugar) and dehydration may result unless you adjust your training.

The main concern is a rise in the mother-to-be's core temperature, especially during the first trimester. During this time a too-high body temperature (hyper-thermia) may cause birth defects. Watch out for overheating and keep your body temperature below 100.4 Fahrenheit, advises the American College of Obstetricians and Gynecologists. To avoid overheating, make sure you:

• Exercise in a cool, ventilated, low-humidity environment

• Drink plenty of cool water

• Practice moderation in intensity and duration.

You need to avoid saunas and hot tubs, too, unless they're set on much lower heat than normal.

Relaxing With Relaxin

Your baby needs space to grow, and thanks to the hormone relaxin and the help of estrogen, he or she will have it! During pregnancy, your ligaments soften, joints loosen, muscles and tendons stretch. Be aware, however, that these changes also make you vulnerable when it

Guidelines for Staying Fit During Pregnancy

As long as your doctor clears you for exercise during your pregnancy, you're good to go. Pay attention to the following recommendations. Some apply to all exercise programs, while others are specific to pregnant athletes.

Weight Training
- Keep in control of the weights.
- Lift and lower the weights in a deliberate manner.
- Maintain good form.
- Stay within a comfortable range of motion.
- Use less weight and more reps. Stick with 3–10-pound weights and 15–20 reps.
- Don't hold your breath on exertion.
- To prevent low blood pressure, don't lie on your back.
- To prevent low-back irritation, avoid lifting over your head.

Stretching
- Stretch muscles that have been warmed up.
- Use static, steady stretches.
- Don't bounce.
- Don't take stretches to maximum resistance.

Aerobic Activity
- Spend more time warming up to increase muscle tem-perature and range of motion (about 10 minutes).
- Stay in your aerobic zone for 15–20 minutes.
- Keep your heart rate below 140 beats per minute.
- Stay with low-impact aerobic-type activity.
- Take your time to cool down (5–10 minutes).

Danger Signals: When It's Time to Stop
Stop immediately if you experience any of the following during exercise:
- Fatigue
- Pain
- Dizziness
- Shortness of breath
- Accelerated heart beat
- Uterine contractions (call your doctor)
- Vaginal bleeding or amniotic fluid leakage (call your doctor).

Additional caveats: Call your doctor if you experience any of the above problems and have been diagnosed with any of the following: high blood pressure, anemia, history of bleeding during pregnancy, problems with placenta or cervix, history of three or more spontaneous abortions, or any diagnosed pre-existing medical condition or high-risk pregnancy.

comes to exercise. Joints may become unstable; posture shifts and muscle imbalances may occur; some muscles tighten and some become weaker. The best thing to do is relax the tight muscles and strengthen the weak ones. Be sure you properly perform stretch and strength exercises.

And remember to breathe as you move through stretches.

'Exercise during pregnancy can lessen fatigue, and improve your mental and emotional outlook.'

Relaxin affects the connective tissue and joints throughout the body, making a pregnant woman more susceptible to joint injury. Never overstretch your muscles; stretch only to the point of feeling it, not to discomfort.

After the 20th week, you may need to modify your stretching and strengthening exercises. No more flat crunches or similar horizontal positions. Lying on your back beyond the first half of pregnancy can cause hypotension because it puts pressure on the inferior vena cava (the large vein carrying blood from the lower body back to the heart). Also avoid

deep-knee bends and overhead exercises. Listen to your body; you'll know.

It's All Good

Research shows that women who exercise experience fewer symptoms and discomforts associated with pregnancy. However, just as you plan your workouts, remember to plan your rest periods too. Clumsiness due to weight gain and shifts, and absentmindedness due to the anticipation of life changes, are part and parcel of pregnancy. Enjoy your pregnancy more by getting plenty of rest and adequate sleep.

77

BACK AFTER BABY

I have always worked out and I definitely think it helped make childbirth easier. Now that I've had my daughter I'd like to start getting back into shape. How long do I have to wait before working out again? Are there any exercises I should avoid?

A: Returning to exercise postpartum is slow going, no matter how much you worked out before you had your baby. Initially, intensity, frequency and duration all take a giant step backward, especially during those first six weeks after your baby is born. Not only has your body just gone through major trauma, but you're now more sleep-deprived than ever and extreme fatigue is an understated way of life. Yet you can start exercising soon after childbirth, as long as you begin gradually, and listen to your body and doctor.

A Time to Heal

"Basically, two areas are affected most after pregnancy: the abdominal muscles and the perineum," states Roscoe Marter, MD, of Valencia, California. "Some women get diastasis during pregnancy, which is where the abdominal wall splits midline." If this occurred, jumping back into abdominal exercises

Easing Down That Road to Fitness

WEEKS 1–2: Rest and recoup, and walk if you're comfortable. Start slowly and don't push yourself at all. If you really feel like you have to do something for your abs, do pelvic tilts on your back; stay away from exercises that directly work your abdominals. And don't forget your Kegels!

WEEKS 3–4: Continue to do pelvic tilts and Kegels. If you don't have diastasis, you can begin to do some crunches, although start very slowly and keep the sets and reps to a minimum, say one or two sets of 10–15. You can begin to do arm and leg work at this time, but stay away from compound exercises such as squats, lunges, etc., and start with very light weight. Choose exercises that offer your body support, preferably seated.

WEEKS 5–6: Continue with the previous weeks' exercises, and slowly add back in those you did prior to childbirth. Be sure to listen to your body, and stop if you're uncomfortable. Also, do light stretches, but be very careful since the hormones in your body make your joints less stable and thus increase the risk of injury.

too soon can further aggravate the condition, and in some cases, cause a hernia-type injury. "During the first two weeks, avoid abdominal exercises, especially crunches," Marter advises. "If you attempt to do crunches and notice a bulge in the [center of your abs], wait a while longer before trying them again." And keep in mind that the belly takes months to return to its former self. The skin, fascia and muscles all need time to tighten back up.

The perineum — the area between the vagina and the rectum — is compromised during a vaginal birth, since most woman often either have episiotomies or tear during their deliveries. This can make even simple tasks, such as sitting and moving your bowels, quite uncomfortable. Allow your body to heal by avoiding straining and doing your Kegel exercises.

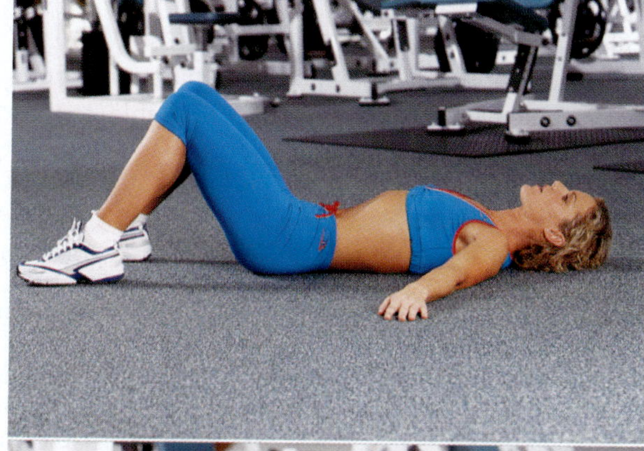

Pelvic tilts are a good exercise to begin with after giving birth.

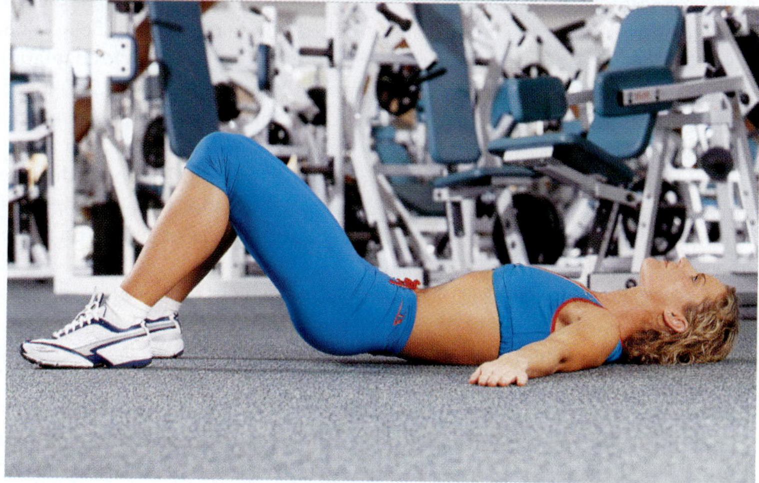

Tips for Breast-Feeding Moms

- "Nurse your baby before your workout," recommends Roscoe Marter, MD, of Valencia, California. "Heavy exercise can cause lactic acid to accumulate in the breastmilk and may alter the taste."
- Don't overdo it; extreme exercise can diminish your milk supply.
- Get plenty of rest, drink lots of fluids and eat healthfully.
- Give yourself a break. Most breast-feeding moms don't drop those last few pounds until their babies are weaned. The body naturally holds on to a little extra bodyfat to ensure a quality milk supply.

A C-section delivery will further limit you. During the first four weeks scarring takes place as the wound heals, so hold off on heavy lifting during this time. Walking, however, is an activity you can do as early as the first day. Just don't walk too fast.

Exercise for Body & Mind

During the postpartum period, women are vulnerable to depression and stress, mostly due to fatigue of having just given birth and caring for a newborn. The psychological benefits of exercise can help you deal with that transition.

You've just experienced one of life's greatest achievements, that of growing and giving birth to another human being. It's no walk in the park physically or emotionally, but the rewards far exceed the challenges of past and future. Congratulations! And don't worry, you will get your body back — just look nine months down the road. ■

References

1. Morio, B., Gachon, A.M., Boirie, Y., et al. Lipolysis, fatness, gender and plasma leptin concentrations in healthy, normal-weight subjects. European Journal of Nutrition 38(1):14–19, 1999.

2. Tarnopolsky, M.A., Bosman, M., Macdonald, J.R., et al. Postexercise protein-carbohydrate and carbohydrate supplements increase muscle glycogen in men and women. Journal of Applied Physiology 83(6):1,877–1,883, 1997.

3. Tarnopolsky, M.A., Atkinson, S.A., Phillips, S.M., MacDougall, J.D. Carbohydrate loading and metabolism during exercise in men and women. Journal of Applied Physiology 78(4):1,360–1,368, 1995.

4. Staron, R.S., Karapondo, D.L., Kraemer, W.J., et al. Skeletal muscle adaptations during early phase of heavy-resistance training in men and women. Journal of Applied Physiology 76(3):1,247–1,255, 1994.

5. Reybrouck, T., Fagard, R. Gender differences in the oxygen transport system during maximal exercise in hypertensive subjects. Chest 115(3):788–792, 1999.

6. Poehlman, E.T., Toth, M.J., Ades, P.A., Calles-Escandon, J. Gender differences in resting metabolic rate and noradrenaline kinetics in older individuals. European Journal of Clinical Investigations 27(1):23–28, 1997.

7. Ettinger, S.M., Silber, D.H., Collins, B.G., et al. Influences of gender on sympathetic nerve responses to static exercise. Journal of Applied Physiology 80(1):245–251, 1996.

8. Marliss, E.B., Kreisman, S.H., Manzon, A., et al. Gender differences in glucoregulatory responses to intense exercise. Journal of Applied Physiology 88(2):457–466, 2000.

9. Elbers, J.M., Asscheman, H., Seidell, J.C., Gooren, L.J. Effects of sex steroid hormones on regional fat depots as assessed by magnetic resonance imaging in transsexuals. American Journal of Physiology 276(2 Pt 1):E317–325, 1999.

10. Kraemer, W.J., Staron, R.S., Hagerman, F.C., et al. The effects of short-term resistance training on endocrine function in men and women. European Journal of Applied Physiology 78(1):69–76, 1998.

11. Barr, S.I., Janelle, K.C., Prior, J.C. Energy intakes are higher during the luteal phase of ovulatory menstrual cycles.

American Journal of Clinical Nutrition 61(1):39–43, 1995.

12. Ebben, W.P., Jensen, R.L. Strength training for women, debunking myths that block opportunity. The Physician & Sportsmedicine 26(5): 86-97, 1998.

13. Fleck, S.J., Kraemer, W.J. Designing resistance training programs. (2nd ed.) Champaign, FL: Human Kinetics, 1997.

14. Lewis, D.A., Kamon, E., Hodgson, J.L. Physiological differences between genders. Sports Medicine 3:357–369, 1986.

15. Cureton, K.J., Collins, M.A., Hill, D.W., McElhannon Jr., F.M. Muscle hypertrophy in men and women. Medicine & Science in Sports & Exercise 20(4):338-344, 1988.

16. O'Hagan, F.T., Sale, D.G., MacDougall, J.D., Garner, S.H. Response to resistance training in young women and men. International Journal of Sorts Medicine (16)5:314-321, 1995.

17. Holloway, J.B., Baechle, T.R. Strength training for female athletes. Sports Medicine 9(4):216–228, 1990.

18. Baechle, T.R. Essentials of strength training and conditioning. National Strength and Conditioning Association. Human Kinetics, 1994.

19. Holloway, J.B., Baechle, T.R. Strength training for female athletes. Sports Medicine 9(4):216–228, 1990.

20. Miskec, C.M., Potteiger, J.A., Nau, K.L., Zebas, C.J. Do varying environmental and menstrual cycle conditions affect aerobic power output in female athletes? Journal of Strength and Conditioning Research 11(4):219–223, 1997.

21. Shangold, M., Mirkin, G. Women and exercise, physiology and sports medicine. FA Davis Company, 1988.

22. American College of Obstetricians and Gynecologists publication AP119, "Exercise During Pregnancy," 1994.

23. Avery, N.D., Stocking, K.D., Tranmer, J.E., et al. Fetal responses to maternal strength conditioning exercises in late gestation. Canadian Journal of Applied Physiology 24(4):362–376, 1999.

24. Hartmann, S., Bung, P. Physical exercise during pregnancy: physiological considerations and recommendations. Journal of Perinatal Medicine 27(3):204–215, 1999.

25. Sternfeld, B. Physical activity and pregnancy outcome. Review and recommendations. Sports Medicine 23(1):33–47, 1997.

26. Stevenson, L. Exercise in pregnancy, part 2: recommendations for individuals. Canadian Family Physician 43(1):107–111, 1997.

INDEX

J

K

L

M

P

Q

R

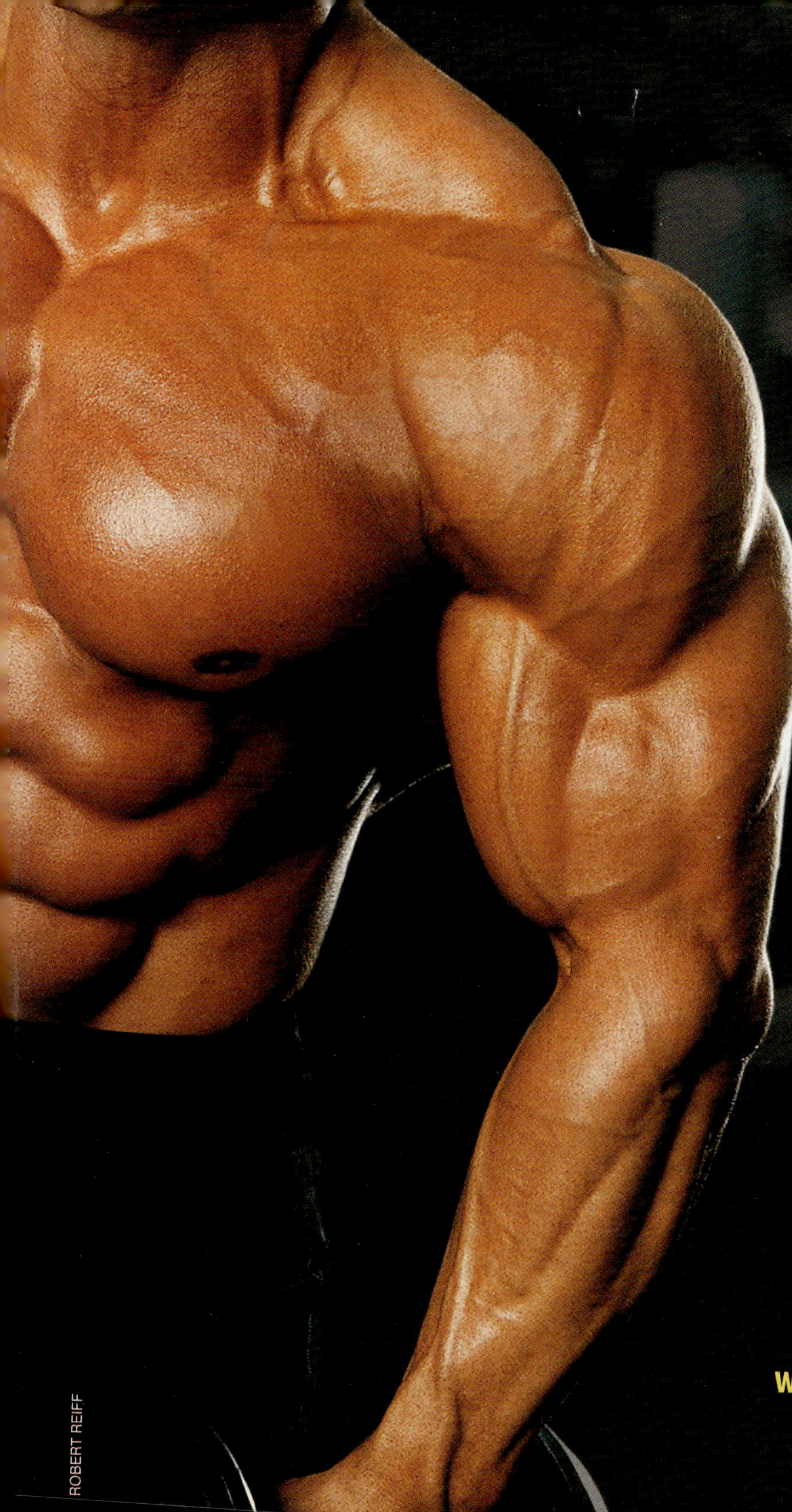
MUSCLE & FITNESS

THE ULTIMATE PERSONAL TRAINER

Subscribe now to MUSCLE & FITNESS and SAVE OVER 55%.*

Maximize your fitness potential with:

- exercise programs for every body part
- nutrition plans & supplement advice to foster muscle growth
- expert tips & techniques for every fitness level

Get the personal training you deserve—call today!

Subscribe NOW & SAVE BIG!

www.muscle-fitnessinfo.com
or call (800) 340-8954

Refer to code V23MSIP. Rates good in U.S. only.
* Savings off the newsstand price.

ROBERT REIFF